# 366 INVENTIVE AND DELICIOUS WAYS TO MAKE YOUR DIET HEALTHY WITH LEAFY GREENS

Our parents always urged us to eat our greens, and now we're doing just that. In today's increasingly health-conscious society, we are more aware than ever that leafy greens are chock-full of vitamins and minerals that are absolutely essential to good health. Linda Romanelli Leahy's flavorful recipes show you how to add leafy greens such as bok choy, dandelion, mesclun, and Swiss chard to your diet for good health and great-tasting meals. In addition to this feast of wonderful recipes, you'll discover in these pages a wealth of useful information:

- An array of cooking methods
- Complete descriptions of more than thirty greens, from arugula to watercress
- Expert advice on selecting, washing, drying, and storing greens
- Nutritional analysis for each recipe

From soup to dessert, this unique volume offers hundreds of new, satisfying ways to healthier eating.

LINDA ROMANELLI LEAHY is a freelance food writer and educator who has written three previous cookbooks. A former editor at *Cooking Light* and *Weight Watchers* magazines, she lives in Bridgehampton, New York.

D1534307

# 366

# Healthful Ways to Cook Leafy Greens

## Linda Romanelli Leahy

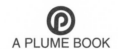

A PLUME BOOK

PLUME
Published by the Penguin Group
Penguin Books USA Inc., 375 Hudson Street,
New York, New York 10014, U.S.A.
Penguin Books Ltd, 27 Wrights Lane,
London W8 5TZ, England
Penguin Books Australia Ltd, Ringwood,
Victoria, Australia
Penguin Books Canada Ltd, 10 Alcorn Avenue,
Toronto, Ontario, Canada M4V 3B2
Penguin Books (N.Z.) Ltd, 182–190 Wairau Road,
Auckland 10, New Zealand

Penguin Books Ltd, Registered Offices:
Harmondsworth, Middlesex, England

First published by Plume, an imprint of Dutton Signet, a division
of Penguin Books USA Inc.

First Printing, June, 1997
10  9  8  7  6  5  4  3  2  1

 REGISTERED TRADEMARK—MARCA REGISTRADA

LIBRARY OF CONGRESS CATALOGING-IN-PUBLICATION DATA:
Leahy, Linda Romanelli.
    366 healthful ways to cook leafy greens / Linda Romanelli Leahy.
        p.   cm.
    Includes index.
    ISBN 0-452-27511-3
    1. Cookery (Greens)   2. Greens, Edible.   I. Title.
TTX803.G74L43   1997
    641.6'54—dc21                                              96-47951
                                                                   CIP

Printed in the United States of America
Set in Garamond Light
Designed by Leonard Telesca

BOOKS ARE AVAILABLE AT QUANTITY DISCOUNTS WHEN USED TO PROMOTE PRODUCTS OR SERVICES. FOR INFORMATION PLEASE WRITE TO
PREMIUM MARKETING DIVISION, PENGUIN BOOKS USA INC., 375 HUDSON STREET, NEW YORK, NEW YORK 10014.

*For Mom and Dad, with love.*

# Acknowledgments

I am always grateful to friends and family for their encouragement whenever I write a book or story or teach a cooking class. Although the work sounds glamorous, many have seen me knee-deep in flour, sans makeup, dressed in a frumpy sweatsuit. On top of this I wrap myself in a huge apron, which by midafternoon is stained with the foods of the day: tomatoes, beets and whatever else needs to be tested. Not a pretty picture but an accurate one. Thank you all, especially:

Corinne Phillips, who kept things organized, edited, washed, chopped, measured, and tested amid jokes and "leafy" language.

Seth Redlus, who spent hours helping me understand a new software program and taking charge when I didn't.

Marie Simmons, who listened when I needed an ear, and sent food packages when I was at the computer rather than in the kitchen.

Kate Leahy, who enthusiastically tested recipes and always thought they were wonderful.

Mary Novitsky, who at the eleventh hour gave me great editing advice and made me laugh.

Andrew Ramer, an angel who sent me a beautiful letter of encouragement just when I needed it.

The Group—Camille, Cat, Chani, and Lisa—our work together has been "soul" food.

Lonny Upson, the produce manager at Jerry and David's Red Horse Market in East Hampton. He tracked down difficult-to-find greens when no one else could.

David Morales, for formatting the table for the greens chart.

The taste-testing crew: Steve Brender; David Binder; Stuart Spitz; Carol and Robert Andresen; Kathleen and Jim Schwartz; John, Cindy, and Parker Roe; Alice and John Murray; Tom Walters; Leslie Benney; William, Raphaela, Gillian, and Melissa Eckert; Chris Griese; and Elizabeth Yastrzemski.

Faith Hamlin, my agent, who's always on the lookout for a good book and keeps me working.

Julia Moskin and Jennifer Moore, my editors at Dutton.

Most of all, Rob Leahy, who ate enough greens for a lifetime.

# Contents

# Introduction

In the Italian-American neighborhood in Brooklyn where I grew up, I used to pick dandelion greens in the vacant lots across the street from my home. These wild greens went into Grandma's salad bowl at dinner. She lived downstairs from us, and ate her dandelion salad alone, because we kids wouldn't eat "weeds." She also wanted us to eat escarole on Mondays, because she believed that they cleaned out your system after Sunday dinner, always an over indulgent marathon meal. We poked around that pot of greens every Monday, but were still reluctant to sample it. Occasionally, broccoli di rape (broccoli raab) appeared at the table, but we would have none of it. The peppery and pungent flavor was just too much for our young and unsophisticated palates.

Mom had her say on the subject, too. She was a spinach advocate, because she said it had lots of iron. My sisters and I didn't much care about iron, but were willing to eat spinach because it helped Popeye heroically save Olive Oyl from the clutches of Bluto every week. We baby boomers were part of the new TV generation. Although my brother didn't come along for another fifteen years, he, too, bought into the Popeye spinach myth, flexing his toddler muscles.

Despite our reluctance to try these vegetables, the women in my family were ahead of the times on the "greens" issue. In the last few years, studies have shown the vitamin and mineral content of dark leafy greens to be a powerhouse of nutrients. Although none of us knew that greens were potent antioxidants (cancer-fighting agents), rich in beta-carotene (a precursor to Vitamin A), Vitamins C and E, calcium, potassium and B vitamins, protein and fiber, we all knew that greens were "good" for us. In fact, those straggly dandelions that I picked but scorned are one of the stars of the leafy greens world, along with arugula and radicchio. The restaurant establishment, in love with Italian food, should get major credit for the popularity of these greens, which are in salads on many menus.

Of course, Italians haven't cornered the market on leafy greens. Cabbage, for instance, is a mainstay in German, Polish, Dutch, and Irish cooking. They've prepared dishes with this vegetable that Italians never dreamed of, accompanied by sour cream, pickled fish, and potatoes.

Always popular, Asian cuisine brings us tat soi, bok choy, mizuna, and a variety of exotic cabbages. These ingredients, once available only in Asian neighborhoods, are now available at the local supermarket.

In a classic display of artistic expression, the French turned leafy greens into an art form, not just a food source. This is evident in the use of leafy greens to wrap fish or terrines or as chiffonade, a French word meaning "made of rags," and in this case these elegant rags consist of thinly shredded sorrel and lettuce used as garnish for soups. We can also thank the French for the term "mesclun," the popular salad mixture of colorful, wild, baby lettuces and other greens.

Within our own borders, we have the Deep South to thank for collards, mustard and turnip greens, and kale. Although these greens used to be boiled to death with a hunk of salt pork added for flavor, even in the South food has lightened up and is being prepared in more nutritious ways.

The world of greens is rich in variety, taste, texture, and nutrients. This book contains recipes using over 35 different types of leafy greens. If you've been a naysayer to leafy greens, but are becoming curious, read on.

**Fresh vs. frozen:** While there are no more empty lots in Brooklyn that have been untouched by urban pollution, dandelions as well as plenty of other wild greens that were once unavailable at the market are now quite common at the supermarket. Most fresh greens tend to be sandy, so if you don't have the time or patience to properly wash them, then I suggest using frozen greens (which are parboiled before packaging) and supplementing your diet with lots of fresh mesclun or spring mixes for salads. These don't need washing.

Frozen greens are a snap to cook in the microwave—you don't even need to remove the packaging. Just the place the box on a microwave-safe dish and cook according to package directions. If your recipe calls for "squeezed" greens, remove the wrapper after cooking and wring the entire package between your hands, over a sink or bowl. This method is a little messy, but easy and effective.

**Selecting greens:** Greens should be just that: green (or red), not yellow. Yellow or brown is a sure sign they're over the hill. Look for bunches with crisp leaves, free from insect holes and bites. Be sure the stems aren't shriveled, because that part is edible too.

**Washing greens:** Not all greens are created equal. Some, depending on the soil in which they're grown, are definitely dirtier and sandier than others, therefore they'll need repeated washing. The following methods are very effective for washing gritty greens:

1. *If you have a double sink,* fill one part with cold water and add the greens. Swirl them around to loosen the dirt, then let them stand about 10 minutes until the grit settles to the bottom. Carefully lift the greens out of the water and put them into the second sink. Drain the water and grit from the first sink. Refill with cold water and repeat the procedure until all the greens are clean.
2. *If you only have one sink,* place the greens in a large colander and run under water for a minute or two. Leave the colander in the sink, then fill the sink with cold water. Let the colander stand a few minutes, then lift it up and drain the water and grit from the sink. Repeat the procedure until all the greens are clean.
3. *Salad spinner method:* Fill the spinner (if it has a solid bottom) with water and place the greens in the strainer insert. Let it stand a few minutes, then lift the insert out and discard the water and grit. Repeat the procedure until all the greens are clean. If your salad spinner is too small, a large bowl and a colander that fits into it will work the same way.

**Storing greens:** Washed greens can last anywhere from 3 to 7 days in the refrigerator depending on the type of leaf. Head lettuce lasts longer than arugula and cabbage, and can actually last for weeks.

After greens are washed, shake the leaves to remove any excess water. Wrap the still wet leaves in dry paper towels and place in a large sealable plastic bag but leave the bag open. Place the bag in the vegetable bin of the refrigerator. After using the greens, rinse out the bag; it's reusable.

There are also perforated plastic bags on the market designed just for vegetables.

**Drying greens:**

1. *Salad spinner:* There are a few different types of salad spinners on the market. I prefer the one with a solid bottom and a pull cord. I have friends, however, who use a spinner with a perforated bottom. This type allows the water to run through the greens and out the bottom into the sink as they spin dry.
2. *The pillowcase method:* This is a great method for people who can't bear the thought of buying yet another gizmo to cram into their already overcrowded cabinets. Just place the washed greens inside the pillowcase and shake vigorously until the pillowcase is wet but the greens aren't.
3. *The toque method:* A friend suggested this method to me years ago, and I've found it very useful. After culinary school, I used my chef's outfit as a Halloween costume (since I didn't choose to work in a restaurant). However, I kept the toque (chef's hat), in my kitchen as a cover for my coffee thermos. It works just like the pillowcase method, but with a little more panache!

## About the Recipes

Here are various definitions for the cooking terms used throughout this book.

**Chiffonade:** Leafy vegetables, classically lettuce and sorrel, cut into very thin strips by stacking and tightly rolling the leaves, then slicing across them.

**Cube:** To cut food in cube-shaped pieces, usually about 1 inch in diameter.

**Dice:** To cut into tiny cubes about ¼ inch in size.

**Dredge:** To coat food lightly with flour or bread crumbs.

**Drizzle:** To pour a thin stream of liquid, often oil, lightly over food. I recommend an oil can with a long, thin spout. It's perfect for drizzling.

**Grill:** This term is used frequently for a number of ways to cook food. Grilling may done on a rack over hot coals, on a rack over gas heat, or on a ridged stovetop grill. This term is also interchangeable with barbecuing and broiling.

**Julienne:** Uniform vegetable strips, cut about ⅛ inch thick and 2 inches long.

**Knead:** The process of manipulating dough mechanically or by hand to form it into a workable mass. The dough is first pressed with the heels of the hands and pushed away from the body. Next it is folded in half toward you, then it is given a quarter turn. The procedure is repeated until the dough is smooth and elastic. This usually takes from 8 to 10 minutes. Kneading may also be done in a food processor or a heavy-duty electric mixer. More information on kneading dough is in the preface to Chapter 10.

**Mince:** To cut food into tiny pieces, about ⅛ inch thick. Minced is smaller than chopped, but the term is interchangeable with finely chopped. I often refer to minced onion (which is raw, not dried) and minced herbs.

**Pinch:** The amount of a dry ingredient you can hold between your thumb and forefinger.

**Poach:** To cook food gently in simmering liquid. This is often the preferred method for cooking foods in order to retain their shape.

**Puree:** Finely mashed food. The easiest way to puree is in a food processor, but pushing food through a sieve or using a food mill will also work.

**Simmer:** To cook food in liquid just below the boiling point. Bubbles will form slowly and break under the surface of the liquid.

**Squeezed:** In this book the term refers to greens, fresh or frozen, which have been cooked, then squeezed, by hand, of excess liquid. If the greens must be very dry, recipe instructions will recommend placing greens in a clean kitchen towel and squeezing again until most of the moisture is removed.

## Methods for Cooking Greens

**Blanch:** To briefly immerse greens in rapidly boiling water, then plunge them into cold water to stop the cooking. With this method, greens will retain their bright color.

**Braise:** To brown meats and vegetables in a small amount of fat, then cook, tightly covered, in a small amount of flavored liquid for a long time over low heat.

**Sauté:** To cook food quickly, in fat, over high heat.

**Steam:** To steam, place the greens in a steamer basket set over simmering water in a wide, tightly covered saucepan. An excellent method for retaining most of the leafy green's nutrients.

**Stir-fry:** To cook small pieces of food quickly in a large pan (usually a wok) in a small amount of very hot fat over high heat. The food is stirred constantly and the method results in crisp, yet tender, texture.

**Wilt:** To wilt, first rinse the leaves, then place the wet leaves in a pot or skillet over low heat and cover tightly. A method in which greens become limp and pliable.

## About Ingredients:

**Balsamic Vinegar:** Italian vinegar produced in the provinces of Modena and Reggio in Northern Italy. It is made from the concentrated juice of white grapes and is aged in barrels, like wine. Authentic "balsamico" is aged a minimum of twelve years and is very expensive. The cheaper brands, which may or may not be from Modena or Reggio, are an excellent choice for marinades.

**Beans:** Dried beans must always be soaked in water overnight, drained and covered with water again before cooking. Check package instructions for a quick soaking method. Canned beans may be substituted. To use, place them in a colander and rinse under cold water. Unrinsed canned beans may be used as a thickener for a soup or stew.

**Bread crumbs:** Dried bread crumbs are best bought in an Italian bakery. They are inexpensive and have no added chemicals. To make your own, preheat the oven to 200 degrees. Place the leftover scraps of either white or whole wheat bread on a baking sheet and bake until the bread is completely dry. Store the bread in a sealed container. When ready to use, grind in a blender or food processor. Place the leftover crumbs in a sealed container and refrigerate or freeze in a sealable plastic bag.

**Broth:** Many recipes call for chicken or vegetable broth. Homemade broth is recommended, but if you use canned broth, I suggest using low-sodium broth to prevent oversalting the food.

**Capers:** Capers are usually sold in jars and are preserved in salt or vinegar and should be rinsed before using. Until my first visit to Italy, however, I had no idea what a fresh caper looked like. There, caper plants grow wild in the chinks of old walls. Although the pink and white flowers of this plant are beautiful, it's the bud that is valued and becomes that little caper we find in jars.

**Cheeses:** A good rule of thumb when considering the fat content in cheese is that the harder the cheese, the lower the fat grams per ounce. Parmigiano-Reggiano and Pecorino Romano cheese are very low in fat, while a creamy cheese, such as mascarpone, is very high. Blue-veined cheeses, although high in fat, are so intense in flavor that a small amount can really perk up a dish.

**Crostini:** These appetizers are small toasted slices of Italian bread spread with a variety of savory toppings. Crostini also double as croutons for soup.

**Egg Substitute:** Personally I think a real egg is one of nature's perfect foods, but if you have a cholesterol problem or are trying to cut down on the fat in your diet, egg substitutes are an alternative. One-quarter cup of egg substitute is equal to one large egg or 2 egg whites.

**Extra-Virgin Olive Oil:** This is the finest grade of olive oil. It is low in acid and fruity in flavor, the result of the first pressing of the olives in which no chemical solvents are used. It is expensive, and I don't recommend it for cooking. It's terrific drizzled over cooked greens and salads.

**Flat-Leaf Parsley:** This herb is often called Italian parsley, because it's used so much in Italian cooking. It is more flavorful than curly-leaf parsley which is often used as a garnish, rather than an ingredient.

**Garam Masala:** This is a blend of ground spices, such as coriander, cinnamon, cardamom, cloves, cumin, and black pepper which produces a hot spicy flavor. Garam Masala is to Indian cuisine what olive oil is to Mediterranean cooking.

**Jicama:** This large, bulbous root vegetable resembles water chestnuts in texture. Its nutty flavor is accented when eaten raw, but jicama may also be cooked.

**Nuts:** Nuts are generally high in fat. Peanuts, however, are a legume (a seeded pod) and are considered a protein. They are high in fat (mostly monounsaturated) but also high in fiber.

A tablespoon or two of any chopped nut used as a garnish adds flavor, eye appeal, and a little crunch to a dish without adding too much fat.

**Olives:** The variety of fresh olives available in stores seems endless. They come in all shapes, sizes, and colors. My favorite are the Greek Kalamata olives. They have an intense salty flavor.

To pit fresh olives, place a few at a time on a large cutting board. Place the blade of a large chef's knife flat on top of the olives; with the heel of your hand press down on the knife. This should squash the olives enough to allow the pits to be removed easily.

**Rind:** The skin of citrus fruits including the white pithy underneath portion.

**Zest:** The brightly colored outer layer of citrus rind (usually from lemons, limes, and oranges), which contains aromatic oils that flavor food. The zest is obtained by using a vegetable peeler or a tool called a zester. In a pinch, a paring knife may be used.

## The Greens

**Arugula (rocket, rucola):** A pungent, tender salad green with a sharp peppery mustard flavor.

**Beet greens:** A form of chard, these slightly sweet and mild-flavored greens may be used raw as well as cooked.

**Belgian endive:** The blanched (a special growing technique) root of chicory. It is 4 to 6 inches long and has a tightly packed, cream-colored head of slightly bitter leaves.

**Bok choy:** A popular variety of Chinese cabbage. Its wide white stalks resemble a celery that flowers into dark leaves. The leaves are mild-tasting; the stalks add crunch to stir-fries.

**Broccoli raab (broccoli di rape, rape, rapini):** This green is also known as bitter broccoli because of its pungent and acrid flavor. It's related to both the cabbage and the turnip family. Its bitter flavor, prized by Italians, is gaining popularity in America.

**Brussels sprouts:** A miniature member of the cabbage family.

**Cabbage (red and green):** These popular varieties come in compact heads and have been cultivated for over 2500 years.

**Chinese cabbage:** Chinese celery cabbage and napa cabbage, in addition to bok choy, are the most widely used Chinese cabbages on the American market. Unlike bok choy, they have crinkly light whitish-green leaves on thick stems. There is more stem than leaf. They, too, are mild tasting.

**Savoy cabbage:** Considered by many to be superior to the red and green variety. Its crinkled leaves are loosely packed and very tender.

**Chicory:** Crisp, curly, sturdy, bitter-tasting green leaves. This family includes escarole, endive and radicchio.

**Curly endive (frisee):** Closely related to chicory. It is a loose head consisting of spiky, light-green-edged outer leaves. The interior heart is almost white, very tender, and slightly less pungent in flavor.

**Collards:** This close relative of kale has dark green, broad, flat leaves. The younger the collards and the thinner the stem, the sweeter they will taste.

**Dandelion:** These have jagged-edged leaves and a tangy, slightly bitter taste. Previously a wild weed, dandelion is now cultivated. Young dandelions have smaller leaves and a less bitter flavor.

**Escarole:** Another member of the chicory family, it is the mildest flavored of that group. It has broad, pale green leaves that are slightly curled. When it is young and tender, it's a delicious addition to the salad bowl.

**Frisee:** See Curly endive.

**Kale:** A member of the cabbage family, kale actually has a faint cabbage flavor. Its frilly, dark blue-green leaves can be pretty tough, but are tender and sweet when cooked properly. It's the green that is often used by caterers to garnish platters.

**Lettuce:** There are four varieties, which are classified as follows:

**Butterhead:** which includes Boston or Bibb. These are tender, leafy heads with a delicate texture.

**Crisphead:** Iceberg is the most popular in this category.

**Leaf:** this variety is often known as looseleaf lettuce. There is no real head, but the leaves are joined at the base. The most popular are red and green leaf lettuce and oak-leaf. These lettuces have tender leaves.

**Romaine (cos):** This is a long-leafed cylindrical lettuce with crunchy ribs. The leaves, usually green, can be tinged with red. It has good texture, like iceberg, but more vitamins and minerals.

**Mache:** This green has many names—field salad, lamb's lettuce, lamb's quarters, and, more commonly, corn salad, because it grows wild in corn fields across the country. The small, tender, piquant leaves of this dark green plant are usually found in "gourmet" salad mixes. Occasionally, mache is sold separately, and may be steamed to make a very tasty side dish.

**Mesclun:** A popular salad mixture of baby lettuces and other miniature greens like orach, red and white Russian kale, red chard, mache, and Asian mustard. Each mixture varies, depending on the producer.

**Mizuna:** A mustard green that can be found in mesclun, although it's being sold separately. It is mild-flavored with decorative dark green, serrated leaves. In Japan it is used as a soup green.

**Mustard greens:** A close relative of the cabbage family, this green has a tangy mustard, pepper flavor. Its bright green leaves are wispier looking than other "Southern" greens like collards or kale, but the older it is, the tougher it gets and the stronger it tastes.

**Radicchio:** The most colorful member of the chicory family. Once unknown in the United States, radicchio is now common. Its burgundy-red leaves and white ribs add great color and bite (it has a strong bitter flavor) to a salad.

**Sorrel (sourgrass):** Sourgrass is a great name for this lemony, tart-tasting herb. The arrow-shaped leaves range from light to dark green. There are different varieties of sorrel, some mellower tasting than others.

**Spinach:** The Spanish are responsible for bringing spinach to our shores. Popeye gets the prize for making it wildly popular. Spinach is an easy green to eat; it's tender, tasty, and colorfully appealing. Most of us think of spinach as a crinkly-leafed green that comes in a cellophane bag. Fresh, farm-grown spinach, a flat, tender-leafed European variety, is far superior.

**Swiss chard (red and green):** A member of the beet family, chard is a green cultivated for its leaves. Unlike beets, it doesn't develop a swollen root. Green chard has a mellower flavor than red, but lacks its beautiful scarlet stems and veins.

**Tat soi:** Although a member of the Chinese cabbage family, tat soi resembles a miniature, glossy green chard leaf. Its flavor, however, is more like arugula or watercress.

**Turnip greens:** There are two types: the young tender tops of turnips and those grown solely for the leaves, which do not form a root ball. Both are slightly sweet when young.

**Watercress:** Another green from the mustard family. Its tiny green leaves pack a sharp peppery flavor. It's sold in small bunches, but occasionally can be found growing wild.

## Yields

The following chart is an approximation of leafy greens cup yields, loosely packed and packed. These measurements were obtained by trimming the vegetables—that is, cutting 1 to 2 inches from the stems or trimming the base in the case of head-type greens like cabbage or bok choy. The greens were then coarsely chopped or shredded and measured. A true measure is impossible, because the amount of stem cut off and discarded is a matter of personal preference. Also, greens lose water as they age and limper bunches will yield less volume.

| LEAFY GREENS: APPROXIMATE YIELDS | | |
|---|---|---|
| Arugula | 1 bunch (6 oz.) | 5 cups loosely packed<br>2 cups packed |
| Beet greens | 1 bunch (1 lb.) | 15 cups loosely packed<br>8 cups packed |
| Bok choy | 1 head (1lb.), with stems | 8 cups loosely packed<br>5 cups packed |
| Broccoli raab | 1 bunch (1¼ lb.) | 14 cups loosely packed<br>9 cups packed |
| Brussels sprouts | 10 oz. | 3 cups |
| Cabbage (red and green) | 1 lb. | 4 to 5 cups |
| Savoy Cabbage | 1 lb. | 9 cups loosely packed<br>6 to 7 cups packed |
| Chinese Cabbage | 1 lb. | 7 cups loosely packed<br>4 to 5 cups packed |
| Chicory | 1 head (1 lb.) | 16 cups loosely packed<br>8 cups packed |
| Collards | 1 bunch (1 lb.), stems removed | 8 cups loosely packed<br>6 cups packed |

| | | |
|---|---|---|
| Curly endive (frisee) | 8 oz. | 4 cups loosely packed<br>2 cups packed |
| Dandelion | 1 bunch (1 lb.) | 8 cups loosely packed<br>4 cups packed |
| Endive | 1 medium head (4 oz.), sliced | 2 cups |
| Escarole | 1 head (1 lb.) | 12 to 13 cups loosely packed<br>8 cups packed |
| Kale | 1 bunch (1 lb.) | 15 to 16 cups loosely packed<br>8 cups packed |
| Mesclun | 4 oz. | 8 cups loosely packed<br>4 cups packed |
| Mizuna | 4 oz. | 8 cups loosely packed<br>4 cups packed |
| Mustard greens | 1 bunch (1 lb.) | 8 cups loosely packed<br>4 to 5 cups packed |
| Radicchio | 1 head (4 oz.) | 3 cups loosely packed<br>2 cups packed |
| Spinach | 1 bag (10 oz.) | 15 cups loosely packed<br>10 cups packed |

| Sorrel | 1 bunch (1lb.) | 8 cups loosely packed<br>5 cups packed |
| --- | --- | --- |
| Swiss chard | 1 bunch (1 lb.) | 10 cups loosely packed<br>5 cups packed |
| Tat soi | 1 bunch (¾ lb.) | 8 cups loosely packed<br>4 cups packed |
| Turnip greens | 1 bunch (1 lb.) | 14 cups loosely packed<br>10 cups packed |
| Watercress | 1 bunch (6 oz.) | 3 cups loosely packed<br>2 cups packed |

# 1
# Soups and Stews

Soup, that steamy satisfying concoction so many of us take for granted, can historically trace its origin to porridge, a grainy, thick mixture. The English "sop" that followed was made by pouring broth over slices of bread. Soon after, anything was fair game (literally) for that pot of broth—meat, poultry, vegetables, fish, grains, legumes, and leafy greens.

The mystical allure of soup is legendary. Unlike the hags of yesteryear, we modern-day cooks don't boil toads and twigs in steaming cauldrons, all the while calling on dark powers to invoke spells and curses. Instead, we add a retired hen, a few vegetables, and a handful of herbs to our pot and call on the magic of chicken soup to cure our complaints and soothe our souls.

Stews, on the other hand, are like a pair of sturdy old shoes. They're comfortable, unsophisticated, and predictable. They promise no cures and hold no surprises. They are hearty, and although thicker than soups, they are not quite porridgelike in consistency. Stewing is a slow-cooking process used to tenderize tougher cuts of meats and stringy or hard vegetables. This method helps release the natural juices of the ingredients and allows flavors to develop and blend.

## Helpful Hints for Making Soups and Stews

1. Broth: Homemade vegetable or chicken broth is preferable to canned, but I realize it's not always possible to prepare broth from scratch. A good alternative is canned low-sodium broth. Most of the time I call for broth by the cup. If a recipe lists 1½ cups (12 ounces) and you're using canned broth, it's OK to use the whole 13¾-ounce can. An additional ounce or two will not spoil the soup.

2. Salt: Most recipes, unless they are water-based, will recommend salt to taste, since the amount needed depends on the type of broth that you use.

3. Leafy greens: Greens cook down quickly and add color, texture, and nutrients to soups and stews. Chopped greens are usually added during the last 15 minutes of cooking. They can be plopped on top of the other ingredients and covered, so that they can steam. A few minutes before cooking time is completed, stir the greens deep into the pot to mix with the other ingredients. Occasionally, raw greens are added or used as a garnish and come to the table in their unadorned, whole, vitamin-packed state.

4. Equipment: A hand blender is a terrific tool for pureeing soups right in the pot with no mess. It's easy to clean too. Just swish it in soapy water to remove food particles, then rinse it in warm water. A regular blender or food processor may be substituted, but isn't as efficient.

# Vegetable Stock

*This makes a lovely pink, slightly sweet stock.*

16 ounces garden salad mix (iceberg lettuce, carrot, and red cabbage)
2 medium ripe tomatoes, quartered
1 red onion, quartered
1 fennel bulb, coarsely chopped

1 rib celery, halved
4 parsley sprigs
1 large garlic clove, mashed
1 bay leaf
1 whole clove
Salt

1. Combine all of the ingredients except the salt with 3 quarts cold water in a stockpot. Bring to a boil over high heat. Reduce the heat and simmer, uncovered, 1 hour. Cool. Strain the stock and discard the solids. Add the salt to taste.

2. Refrigerate up to one week or freeze in 1-, 2-, or 4-cup containers depending on how you intend to use them.

MAKES 10 CUPS

**Variation:** This is a tasty broth made from vegetable trimmings. You can use any veggies ready to go over the hill but not quite there yet. Combine 2 cups spinach stems and trimmings (or any other nonbitter leafy green), 1 coarsely chopped leek (green part only), celery tops, 2 coarsely chopped, trimmed carrots, and 2 sprigs marjoram in a large pot. Add 6 cups water. Bring to a boil over high heat; reduce the heat and follow the above instructions.

Kilocalories 28 Kc • Protein 1 Gm • Fat 0 Gm • Percent of calories from fat 7% • Cholesterol 0 mg • Dietary Fiber 2 Gm • Sodium 20 mg • Calcium 28 mg

# Scotch Broth with Kale

*This is a wonderful winter soup. For a vegetarian soup, eliminate the chicken and use onion bouillon.*

1 tablespoon olive oil
½ cup chopped onion
  (1 medium)
1 garlic clove, minced
1 boneless, skinless chicken
  breast (8 ounces), cut into
  1-inch cubes
2 cups (packed) coarsely
  chopped kale
1 cup cubed pared turnip
½ cup frozen green baby lima
  beans

½ cup cubed pared butternut
  squash
½ cup sliced pared parsnips
¼ cup golden raisins
¼ cup medium barley
2 cubes chicken bouillon or 1
  tablespoon granules
1 bay leaf
1 teaspoon crushed dried thyme
1 can (19 ounces) drained
  chickpeas or 2 cups fresh,
  cooked

1. Heat the oil in a Dutch oven over medium-high heat. Add the onion and garlic and cook 2 minutes, stirring frequently. Add the chicken and cook 3 to 5 minutes until browned on all sides.

2. Stir in 5 cups water and all of the remaining ingredients except the chickpeas. Bring to a boil. Reduce the heat and simmer, covered, 1 hour, adding more water if necessary. Add the chickpeas and cook, uncovered, 15 minutes longer. Remove the bay leaf before serving.

SERVES 4

Kilocalories 407 Kc • Protein 29 Gm • Fat 9 Gm • Percent of calories from fat 19%
• Cholesterol 48 mg • Dietary Fiber 12 Gm • Sodium 971 mg • Calcium 145 mg

# Chilled Lettuce Soup

1 tablespoon unsalted butter
½ tablespoon vegetable oil
1 cup sliced leek, white part only
1 medium shallot, minced
4 cups vegetable broth or
  water
1 package (10 ounces) salad mix
  (romaine and leaf lettuce),
  finely chopped

3 medium potatoes, pared and
  diced (about 2½ cups)
Salt
Freshly ground pepper
1 tablespoon snipped fresh dill
3 tablespoons half-and-half

1. Melt the butter in a Dutch oven over medium heat. Add the oil, leek, and shallot; toss to coat. Cover and cook 2 minutes until the leeks are softened.

2. Add the broth, salad mix, and potatoes. Cook, partially covered, until the potatoes are tender, about 15 minutes. Season with salt and pepper to taste and stir in the dill. Cool, then refrigerate at least 3 hours.

3. Before serving, stir in the half-and-half.

SERVES 4

Kilocalories 236 Kc • Protein 6 Gm • Fat 6 Gm • Percent of calories from fat 24% • Cholesterol 12 mg • Dietary Fiber 4 Gm • Sodium 112 mg • Calcium 72 mg

# Squash Soup with Broccoli Raab Croutons

1 tablespoon unsalted butter
1 cup finely chopped onion
2 cups chopped, seeded, pared
   butternut squash
5 medium yellow summer squash,
   sliced
3 cups chicken broth
Salt

Freshly ground pepper
1 tablespoon olive oil
1 cup chopped broccoli raab
   (leaves only)
4 thin slices French baguette,
   toasted
Kosher or coarse salt

1. Melt the butter in a Dutch oven over medium heat; add the onion and cook about 3 minutes, until soft, stirring occasionally.

2. Add the butternut and yellow squash, stirring to coat. Cover, and cook 2 minutes. Uncover and cook 2 minutes longer, stirring frequently.

3. Add the broth and bring to a boil. Reduce the heat and simmer, partially covered, until the squash is tender, about 20 minutes. Season with salt and pepper to taste. Cool slightly and puree the soup, in batches, in a food processor or blender. Return to the pot and warm over low heat.

4. Meanwhile, heat the oil in a medium skillet or wok over high heat. When the oil is smoking, add the broccoli raab. Cook about 2 minutes or until crisp, stirring frequently. Top each piece of toasted baguette with the greens and sprinkle with a pinch of kosher salt. Ladle the soup into 4 bowls. Garnish each with a slice of toast and serve immediately.

SERVES 4

Kilocalories 263 Kc • Protein 8 Gm • Fat 10 Gm • Percent of calories from fat 32%
• Cholesterol 11 mg • Dietary Fiber 6 Gm • Sodium 240 mg • Calcium 180 mg

# Creole Chicken and Collards

*Creole cooking reflects the cultural and ethnic diversity of New Orleans. Originally a French butter- and cream-based cuisine, it eventually adapted African and Spanish ingredients as well. This Louisiana-style stew is great with corn bread or grilled polenta.*

1½ tablespoons vegetable oil

1¼ pounds boneless, skinless chicken thighs, cut into 1½-inch pieces

1 cup small, whole fresh or frozen peeled onions

1 cup coarsely chopped green bell pepper

½ cup chopped celery

2 ounces chopped turkey or meatless bacon

2 garlic cloves, crushed

2 cups chopped fresh collard greens

1½ cups canned whole peeled tomatoes with juice

1 cup fresh or frozen corn kernels

½ teaspoon salt

¼ teaspoon freshly ground pepper

2 cups (about 8 ounces) fresh okra, trimmed

1. Heat the oil in a Dutch oven over medium heat; add the chicken, onions, green pepper, celery, bacon, and garlic. Cook 5 minutes, stirring frequently. Add the collards and cook 3 minutes longer.

2. Add 1½ cups water, the tomatoes, corn, salt, and pepper; cover and simmer 1 hour, adding more water if necessary. Add the okra and cook 30 minutes longer.

SERVES 4

Kilocalories 488 Kc • Protein 46 Gm • Fat 22 Gm • Percent of calories from fat 40% • Cholesterol 140 mg • Dietary Fiber 7 Gm • Sodium 615 mg • Calcium 243 mg

# Louisiana Catfish Gumbo

*Gumbo, a Cajun specialty from the Bayou country of Louisiana, is a stew with two essential ingredients: okra and filé powder, a spice made from dried, ground sassafras leaves.*

1 tablespoon vegetable oil
1 yellow bell pepper, seeded and
  coarsely chopped
½ cup chopped celery
1 can (14½ ounces) coarsely
  chopped canned tomatoes
  with juice
1 pound (about 2 cups) fresh
  okra, trimmed, or one package
  (10 ounces) frozen okra

1 cup chopped fresh mustard
  greens
1 cup sliced scallions
1 cup vegetable broth
½ teaspoon salt
1 pound catfish fillets,
  cut into 1×1½-inch
  pieces
1 teaspoon gumbo filé powder

Heat the oil in a Dutch oven over medium-high heat. Cook the pepper and celery 5 minutes, stirring frequently. Add the tomatoes, okra, greens, scallions, broth, and salt; reduce the heat to medium and simmer 15 minutes. Add the catfish and cook 15 minutes longer, or until the fish is opaque and tender. Sprinkle each serving with ¼ teaspoon filé powder and serve immediately.

SERVES 4

Kilocalories 212 Kc • Protein 22 Gm • Fat 7 Gm • Percent of calories from fat 30% • Cholesterol 66 mg • Dietary Fiber 3 Gm • Sodium 403 mg • Calcium 97 mg

# Pasta, Spinach and Cauliflower Soup

2 teaspoons olive oil
½ cup diced carrot
¼ cup finely chopped
    onion
2 cups cauliflower florets
1 cup small spinach pasta shells
    (about 3 ounces)

1 tablespoon chopped fresh basil
    (1 teaspoon dried)
½ teaspoon salt
2 cups chopped fresh spinach
1 tablespoon grated Romano
    cheese
Freshly ground pepper

Heat the oil in a large saucepan over medium-high heat. Cook the carrot and onion 5 minutes or until tender, stirring occasionally. Add the cauliflower and 4 cups water. Cover and cook 5 minutes. Stir in the shells, basil, and salt; bring to a boil. Cook 12 to 16 minutes or until the shells are tender; add the spinach during the last 5 minutes of cooking. Sprinkle with the cheese and season with pepper to taste.

SERVES 4

Kilocalories 108 Kc • Protein 5 Gm • Fat 3 Gm • Percent of calories from fat 27% • Cholesterol 2 mg • Dietary Fiber 3 Gm • Sodium 358 mg • Calcium 77 mg

# Spring Pea Soup

*Celebrate the season with this lovely, light soup. Fresh mint is preferable to dried in this recipe.*

1 tablespoon unsalted butter
½ cup chopped onion
1 tablespoon all-purpose flour
1½ cups chicken broth
2 cups shelled fresh peas
½ cup (packed) fresh spinach
   leaves
1 tablespoon chopped fresh mint
   leaves (1 teaspoon dried)

1 teaspoon granulated sugar
½ teaspoon curry powder
⅛ teaspoon white pepper
½ teaspoon grated lemon
   zest
⅓ cup 1% milk
2 tablespoons half-and-half
Finely chopped fresh mint for
   garnish, optional

1. Melt the butter in a Dutch oven over medium heat. Cook the onion 5 minutes, until soft. Add the flour and cook 5 minutes.

2. Stir in the broth and 1½ cups water and bring to a boil, stirring frequently. Add the peas, spinach, mint, sugar, curry, and pepper. Simmer 8 to 10 minutes longer; remove from the heat. Let it cool slightly. Stir in the lemon zest.

3. Puree the soup in small batches in a food processor or blender. Return to the Dutch oven; add the milk and half-and-half. Warm over low heat; do not boil. Ladle the soup into serving bowls; sprinkle with mint, if desired.

SERVES 4

Kilocalories 140 Kc • Protein 7 Gm • Fat 6 Gm • Percent of calories from fat 34% • Cholesterol 13 mg • Dietary Fiber 4 Gm • Sodium 58 mg • Calcium 68 mg

# Carrot Soup with Mustard Greens (Microwave)

1 tablespoon unsalted butter
3 garlic cloves, minced
4 cups sliced carrots
6 ounces potatoes, pared and
  sliced
2¼ cups vegetable broth
1 tablespoon honey

1 teaspoon salt
2 teaspoons snipped fresh dill
  (½ teaspoon dried)
2 cups thinly sliced, then coarsely
  chopped, tender young
  mustard greens

1. Combine the butter and garlic in a 3-quart microwave-safe casserole. Microwave on High for 2 minutes.

2. Add the carrots, potatoes, and ¼ cup of the vegetable broth; cover and vent. Microwave on High for 12 to 14 minutes, until the carrots and potatoes are tender, stirring once. Cool slightly. Puree in a food processor or blender.

3. Return the mixture to the casserole and stir in the remaining 2 cups of broth. Cover and microwave on High for 4 to 6 minutes, until it boils.

4. Stir in the honey, salt, and dill. Ladle into soup bowls. Top each serving with ½ cup mustard greens.

SERVES 4

Kilocalories 198 Kc • Protein 4 Gm • Fat 4 Gm • Percent of calories from fat 15% • Cholesterol 8 mg • Dietary Fiber 6 Gm • Sodium 714 mg • Calcium 87 mg

# Turkey Kielbasa Stew

8 ounces fully-cooked turkey
    kielbasa, sliced
4 medium carrots, pared and cut
    into 1½-inch chunks
2 medium potatoes (about 8
    ounces), pared and diced
1 cup shredded red cabbage

1 cup chicken broth
½ cup lentils
1 package (9 ounces) frozen
    Italian green beans
Salt
2 tablespoons snipped fresh
    chives*

1. Combine the kielbasa, carrots, potatoes, cabbage, broth, and lentils with 3 cups water in a Dutch oven, over medium-high heat.

2. Bring to a boil. Reduce the heat, cover, and simmer 20 minutes. Add the frozen green beans and salt to taste; cook 15 minutes longer until the vegetables are tender. Stir in the chives and serve immediately.

SERVES 4

*Dried chives have no flavor. If fresh are unavailable use scallions.

Kilocalories 287 Kc • Protein 19 Gm • Fat 6 Gm • Percent of calories from fat 19%
• Cholesterol 31 mg • Dietary Fiber 13 Gm • Sodium 557 mg • Calcium 75 mg

# Vegetable Soup with Blue Cheese Toast

*Simple and delicious.*

2 teaspoons vegetable oil
1 tablespoon minced, fresh
  ginger
2 cups mixed vegetable juice
2 cups chicken broth
1 cup sliced carrots

1 cup shredded romaine lettuce
½ cup snow peas, cut diagonally
  in thirds
2 slices whole wheat bread
4 ounces blue cheese,
  crumbled

1. Heat the oil over medium-heat in a Dutch oven. Add the ginger and sauté 1 to 2 minutes, stirring frequently. Stir in the vegetable juice, broth, and carrots and bring to a boil. Reduce the heat and simmer, covered, for 30 minutes.

2. Stir the lettuce and snow peas into the soup. Simmer, uncovered, 10 minutes longer, stirring occasionally.

3. Preheat the broiler.

4. Meanwhile, trim the crusts from the bread and place on a baking sheet. Toast on one side, 4 inches from the heat source in the broiler. Remove and quarter each slice diagonally. Mound the untoasted side with blue cheese. Return to the baking sheet and broil for 1 to 2 minutes, until the cheese is bubbly. Ladle the hot soup into bowls and top each with 2 cheese toasts.

SERVES 4

Kilocalories 227 Kc • Protein 11 Gm • Fat 13 Gm • Percent of calories from fat 48%
• Cholesterol 24 mg • Dietary Fiber 4 Gm • Sodium 970 mg • Calcium 198 mg

# Salad Gazpacho Soup

*A more complex flavor develops if this soup is refrigerated overnight.*

1 package (8½ ounces) salad greens (iceberg, Chinese cabbage, and carrot mix or your choice)
3 cups tomato juice
1 cup vegetable broth
4 scallions, sliced (about ½ cup)
2 large ripe tomatoes, chopped
1 medium green bell pepper, seeded and diced

½ cup chopped peeled cucumber
¼ cup red wine vinegar
1 tablespoon olive oil
2 teaspoons Worcestershire sauce
1 teaspoon salt
¼ teaspoon Tabasco sauce
Sliced scallion greens for garnish, optional

1. Chop any large chunks of lettuce. Add the salad greens to a medium saucepan with the tomato juice and broth. Cook over medium-low heat, covered, 15 minutes until the lettuce is wilted. Cool slightly.

2. Place the lettuce mixture in a refrigerator container. Stir in the remaining ingredients except for the optional garnish and cover. Refrigerate 3 hours or overnight. To serve, garnish with scallion, if desired.

SERVES 4

Kilocalories 117 Kc • Protein 4 Gm • Fat 4 Gm • Percent of calories from fat 28% • Cholesterol 0 mg • Dietary Fiber 4 Gm • Sodium 667 mg • Calcium 61 mg

# Winter Cabbage Borscht

*My friend Steve tasted this recipe and declared that it wasn't borscht. His mother never added cabbage to her beet soup. So, I called the Russian Tea Room in New York City, a landmark restaurant famous for its borscht and celebrity clientele, and sure enough, theirs is made with cabbage. I'm sure both versions are bona fide borscht reflecting different parts of Eastern Europe.*

1 cup chopped onion
1 tablespoon vegetable oil
3 cups shredded cabbage
5 cups vegetable broth
1 bunch beets (1½ pounds),
  pared and shredded
1 medium potato, pared and
  diced
1 large carrot, pared and diced

3 tablespoons lemon juice
1 tablespoon sugar
1 bay leaf
2 tablespoons snipped
  fresh dill
Salt and freshly ground pepper
Nonfat sour cream for garnish,
  optional

1. Combine the onion and oil in a Dutch oven. Cover and cook for 3 minutes over medium heat until the onion is softened. Add the cabbage and cook 5 minutes longer, stirring frequently.

2. Add the broth, beets, potato, carrot, lemon juice, sugar, bay leaf, and 2 cups of water. Bring to a boil, reduce the heat, and simmer 30 minutes or until the potato and carrot are tender. Stir in the dill and season with salt and pepper. Remove the bay leaf. Place in soup bowls and garnish with sour cream.

SERVES 6

Kilocalories 164 Kc • Protein 4 Gm • Fat 3 Gm • Percent of calories from fat 14% • Cholesterol 0 mg • Dietary Fiber 5 Gm • Sodium 171 mg • Calcium 48 mg

# Potato Soup with Beet Green Chiffonade

*This is a great first course for company. When the beet greens are swirled into the soup, deep pink streaks appear on the white backdrop—very dramatic. If you prefer your soup richer, use whole milk.*

4 medium potatoes (or about 4 cups, diced)
1 tablespoon unsalted butter
1 cup chopped celery
1 cup chopped onion

1½ teaspoons salt
3 cups 1% milk
4 cups chiffonade of beet greens
Freshly ground pepper

1. Pare and dice the potatoes. Place in a bowl and cover with cold water.

2. Melt the butter in a Dutch oven over medium heat. Add the celery and onion; cook 5 minutes, stirring frequently.

3. Drain the potatoes and add to the pot with the salt and 2 cups water. Cook 10 minutes. Stir in the milk, partially cover, and cook 10 minutes longer or until the potatoes are tender.

4. Cool slightly. Puree the soup in batches in a blender. Return to the pot and heat. Ladle the soup into bowls. Garnish with the beet greens and a sprinkling of pepper.

SERVES 6

Kilocalories 268 Kc • Protein 10 Gm • Fat 4 Gm • Percent of calories from fat 12% • Cholesterol 10 mg • Dietary Fiber 6 Gm • Sodium 811 mg • Calcium 248 mg

# Kale and Two Potato Soup

*The sweet potato is not related to the white potato, but when you combine them you get lots of vitamins: C, A, B-6, and potassium. Kale provides additional Vitamin C and A plus calcium and iron. The best part is that this soup is delicious, not just nutritious.*

2 cups chopped onion
1 small garlic clove, crushed
1 tablespoon vegetable oil
2 cups chicken broth
1 pound sweet potatoes,
    pared and cut into 1-inch cubes

1 pound white russet potatoes,
    pared and cut into 1-inch cubes
2 cups skim milk
4 cups (packed) chopped kale
¼ teaspoon fennel seeds, crushed
Salt and freshly ground pepper

1. Combine the onion, garlic, and oil in a Dutch oven. Cook over medium heat, stirring occasionally until tender, 3 to 5 minutes. Add the broth, 2 cups water, and the potatoes. Bring to a boil. Reduce the heat to medium-low and cook, covered, until the potatoes are tender, about 20 minutes. Cool slightly.

2. Using a slotted spoon, place about half of the potato mixture in the bowl of a food processor and add about half of the cooking liquid. Puree the potatoes until they are smooth. Return to the pot and stir in the milk. Bring to a simmer over medium heat.

3. Add the kale and fennel, reduce the heat to low, cover, and cook 25 minutes. Uncover, stir, and cook 10 minutes longer, or until the kale is tender. Season with salt and pepper and serve.

SERVES 4

Kilocalories 359 Kc • Protein 12 Gm • Fat 6 Gm • Percent of calories from fat 14% • Cholesterol 4 mg • Dietary Fiber 9 Gm • Sodium 149 mg • Calcium 270 mg

# Chicory and White Bean Soup

*I often place a friselle (a hard Italian biscuit) in the bottom of each serving bowl. Friselli are available at most Italian bakeries.*

1 tablespoon olive oil
2 large garlic cloves, minced
1 head chicory (about 1 pound), trimmed and coarsely chopped (wet)
4 cups chicken broth

4 cups cooked small white beans
2 tablespoons chopped fresh tarragon (2 teaspoons dried)
Salt and freshly ground pepper

1. Heat the oil in a Dutch oven over medium heat. Add the garlic and cook for 30 seconds.

2. Add the wet chicory to the pot, cover, and cook 5 minutes, stirring once. Reduce the heat and add the broth, beans, and tarragon.

3. Simmer 10 minutes. Season with salt and pepper to taste and serve.

SERVES 6

Kilocalories 231 Kc • Protein 15 Gm • Fat 5 Gm • Percent of calories from fat 17 % • Cholesterol 3 mg • Dietary Fiber 11 Gm • Sodium 103 mg • Calcium 186 mg

# Very Green Split Pea Soup

*Split pea soup will thicken when not served immediately. Although additional water or broth will thin it out, the flavor will be diluted.*

1 pound dried split peas (about 2½ cups)
1 tablespoon vegetable oil
1 leek (white part only), thinly sliced
1 large garlic clove, minced
4 cups chicken or vegetable broth

½ teaspoon ground cumin
½ teaspoon salt
1 package (10 ounces) fresh spinach, trimmed and coarsely chopped
½ teaspoon freshly ground pepper
½ cup croutons, optional

1. Soak the peas for 30 minutes. Rinse, sort any debris from the peas, and drain.

2. Heat the oil in a Dutch oven over medium heat. Stir in the leeks and cook about 2 minutes, stirring frequently. Stir in the garlic and cook 1 minute longer.

3. Add the drained split peas and broth with 4 cups water to the leek mixture. Bring to a boil over high heat; reduce the heat and simmer 45 minutes or until the peas are tender. Stir in the cumin and salt; top with the spinach. Cover and cook 15 minutes longer, stirring once. Season with the pepper, sprinkle with the croutons, if desired, and serve immediately.

SERVES 4

Kilocalories 526 Kc • Protein 35 Gm • Fat 8 Gm • Percent of calories from fat 13% • Cholesterol 4 mg • Dietary Fiber 34 Gm • Sodium 462 mg • Calcium 161 mg

# Beans and Spinach Provençal

2 cups navy beans, soaked in
   water overnight
2 tablespoons olive oil
2 cups diced onion
2 cups diced celery
6 garlic cloves, minced
8 cups chicken broth
1 can (14 ounces) Italian-style
   tomatoes, chopped and
   drained

1 tablespoon herbes de Provence
   (combination of dried basil,
   fennel seed, marjoram,
   rosemary, sage, and
   thyme)
3 cups coarsely chopped fresh
   spinach
1 teaspoon salt
2 cups small cooked pasta,
   optional

1. Heat the oil in a large Dutch oven over medium heat. Add the onion, celery, and garlic and cook 10 minutes, stirring frequently. Add the broth, tomatoes, herbs, and drained beans. Reduce the heat and simmer, partially covered, for 1½ to 2 hours or until the beans are tender.

2. Stir in the spinach and salt; cook 15 minutes. Add the pasta and cook 2 minutes longer or until heated through.

SERVES 4

**Variation:** Substitute chopped fennel for celery and ½ cup chopped fresh basil for herbes de Provence. You may also use tat soi or Swiss chard instead of spinach.

Kilocalories 578 Kc • Protein 33 Gm • Fat 14 Gm • Percent of calories from fat 21% • Cholesterol 9 mg • Dietary Fiber 31 Gm • Sodium 1129 mg • Calcium 308 mg

# Split Pea, Stewed Tomato, and Collard Soup

2 cups dried split peas
3 tablespoons olive oil
1 rib celery, diced
1 cup diced onion
2 garlic cloves, crushed
1 bay leaf

1 can (15 ounces) stewed tomatoes
4 cups chopped fresh collard greens
½ teaspoon salt
¼ teaspoon freshly ground pepper

1. Soak the peas for 30 minutes. Rinse and remove any pebbles.

2. Heat the oil in a Dutch oven over medium heat. Add the celery, onion, and garlic and cook 5 minutes until softened.

3. Add the split peas, bay leaf, and 8 cups of water. Bring to a boil, reduce the heat, and simmer for 1½ hours.

4. Add the tomatoes, greens, salt, and pepper and cook 15 minutes. Remove the bay leaf before serving.

SERVES 4

Kilocalories 486 Kc • Protein 27 Gm • Fat 12 Gm • Percent of calories from fat 21% • Cholesterol 0 mg • Dietary Fiber 27 Gm • Sodium 889 mg • Calcium 118 mg

# Collard and Corn Chowder

2 tablespoons vegetable oil
½ cup coarsely chopped onion
½ cup diced green bell pepper
1 package (10 ounces) frozen
   chopped collard greens,
   thawed

1 package (10 ounces) frozen
   corn kernels, thawed
1 cup 1% milk
1 cup low-fat buttermilk
½ teaspoon salt
⅛ teaspoon ground red
   pepper

1. Heat the oil in a medium saucepan over medium-high heat. Add the onion and green pepper; cook 3 minutes, stirring occasionally.

2. Add the collards, corn, and milk; reduce the heat and simmer 5 minutes. Stir in the buttermilk, salt, and ground red pepper. Cook 3 minutes or until heated through. Do not boil. Serve immediately.

SERVES 4

Kilocalories 211 Kc • Protein 9 Gm • Fat 8 Gm • Percent of calories from fat 33% • Cholesterol 5 mg • Dietary Fiber 3 Gm • Sodium 428 mg • Calcium 311 mg

# Vegetable Rice Soup

*Friend, cookbook author, and syndicated columnist Marie Simmons graciously shared one of her delicious recipes, which I adapted for this book.*

8 cups chicken broth
4 cups (packed) chopped
   escarole
2 cups diced carrots
⅓ cup uncooked rice
1 cup trimmed and diced yellow
   squash

1 cup diced tomato, fresh or
   canned (without juice)
½ cup peas, fresh or frozen
   (thawed)
Salt and freshly ground pepper
Grated Parmesan cheese,
   optional

1. Heat the broth to boiling in a large saucepan. Add the escarole, carrots, and rice and cook, uncovered, stirring occasionally until the rice and vegetables are tender, about 20 minutes.

2. Add the squash, tomatoes, and peas. Reduce the heat and simmer, uncovered, until tender, about 10 minutes. Season with salt and pepper. Serve sprinkled with cheese, if desired.

SERVES 6

Kilocalories 150 Kc • Protein 7 Gm • Fat 4 Gm • Percent of calories from fat 23% • Cholesterol 6 mg • Dietary Fiber 4 Gm • Sodium 160 mg • Calcium 49 mg

# Spinach Soup with Herb Dumplings

*This is a quick soup for cold days. The dumplings are made in the time it takes for the soup to come to a boil.*

1 tablespoon vegetable oil
½ cup chopped onion
6 cups chicken broth
1 cup (packed) shredded fresh
  spinach
Salt and freshly ground pepper

*Herb Dumplings:*

1 cup Bisquick or low-fat biscuit
  mix
1 cup oat bran
⅔ cup skim milk
½ teaspoon dried dill

1. Heat the oil in a Dutch over medium heat. Add the onion and cook 3 minutes until tender.

2. Add the chicken broth, spinach, salt, and pepper; bring to a boil over medium heat.

3. Combine the Bisquick, oat bran, milk, and dill in a medium bowl. Mix with a fork until a soft dough forms. Drop by rounded tablespoonfuls into the boiling soup. Reduce the heat and cook, uncovered, 10 minutes; cover and cook 10 minutes longer until the dumplings are done.

SERVES 6

Kilocalories 201 Kc • Protein 8 Gm • Fat 9 Gm • Percent of calories from fat 36% • Cholesterol 5 mg • Dietary Fiber 3 Gm • Sodium 362 mg • Calcium 75 mg

# Spinach Soup (Microwave)

1 package (10 ounces) frozen
  chopped spinach
2 tablespoons chopped
  shallots
1 tablespoon unsalted butter

3 tablespoons all-purpose flour
¾ teaspoon salt
⅛ teaspoon freshly ground
  pepper
3 cups skim milk

1. Remove the outer paper wrapping from the package of spinach. Place the package on a paper towel; microwave on High for 3 to 6 minutes, or until the spinach is thawed. Drain well.

2. Combine the shallots and butter in a 2-quart microwave-safe casserole. Microwave, uncovered, on High for 1 to 1½ minutes.

3. Stir in the flour, salt, and pepper. Gradually whisk in the milk until smooth; add the spinach. Microwave on High for 10 to 12 minutes, or until thick and bubbly, stirring 3 times. Serve immediately.

SERVES 4

Kilocalories 133 Kc • Protein 9 Gm • Fat 4 Gm • Percent of calories from fat 23% • Cholesterol 11 mg • Dietary Fiber 2 Gm • Sodium 623 mg • Calcium 338 mg

# Chilled Potato Soup with Belgian Endive

*Cottage cheese is a tasty and low-fat way to thicken soups.*

2 medium potatoes (about 1 pound)
1 tablespoon unsalted butter
2 teaspoons vegetable oil
1 cup sliced leek (white part only)
½ cup sliced celery
2½ cups chicken broth
¼ teaspoon white pepper
¾ cup nonfat cottage cheese
Salt
1 head Belgian endive, thinly sliced, plus additional for garnish, optional

1. Pare and dice the potatoes. Place in a bowl and cover with cold water.

2. Add the butter and oil to a 3-quart saucepan. Melt the butter over medium heat. Add the leek and celery and cook 3 minutes until they are softened, stirring frequently.

3. Drain the potatoes and add to the pot with the broth and pepper. Bring to a boil. Reduce the heat, cover, and simmer until the potatoes are tender, about 20 minutes; cool.

4. Puree the soup and cottage cheese in a blender. Add salt if necessary. Pour into a refrigerator container and stir in the endive. Cover and refrigerate 3 hours. To serve, ladle the soup into bowls and garnish with endive, if desired.

SERVES 4

Kilocalories 218 Kc • Protein 11 Gm • Fat 7 Gm • Percent of calories from fat 29% • Cholesterol 15 mg • Dietary Fiber 3 Gm • Sodium 236 mg • Calcium 67 mg

# 2
# Sensational Salads

**S**alads and I go back a long way. My Mom served salad at every evening meal. To this day, so do I. I can't imagine dinner without a salad course at the end.

Making salad can be a wonderfully creative process. Salads can be a mixture of almost anything you have on hand in the refrigerator—leafy greens combined with bits of poultry, fish, and/or beans; fruit; cheese; olives; and cooked or raw vegetables—the combinations are endless. Mix and match assertive and tender greens to add taste and textural contrast. Use different color greens in the same salad—red, white, and green leaves tossed together are appealing and delicious. Mesclun and the new packaged salad greens eliminate the need for washing and chopping. What could be quicker than drizzling them with a little extra-virgin olive oil and a squeeze of fresh lemon juice?

The basics of salad-making are pretty straightforward: first trim the greens of any browned edges or wilted, soggy leaves (if the entire bunch of greens is slightly wilted, however, a soaking in ice-cold water may bring it back to life). Greens should then be washed and dried thoroughly.

The big question: Should leaves be torn or cut? I usually tear tender leaves, like Boston or Bibb lettuce, and I often use a knife to shred sturdier leaves (romaine, iceberg, chicory). Contrary to popular belief, the cut edges will not turn brown if you serve the salad within an hour or two, especially if you refrigerate the greens, covered with a damp paper towel, until ready to use. Greens may also be snipped with a scissors. I often do this with small bunches of greens, like arugula, dandelion, and watercress. Whether you cut, tear, or snip greens, it is important that the leaves be in bite-size pieces.

If you don't have the particular green called for in a recipe, just use what you have on hand. Be sure though that you use the same amount the recipe calls for, otherwise the dressing may not be enough (or may be too much) to coat the greens.

Salad dressing may be made ahead and refrigerated, but don't dress the salad until just before serving or it will get soggy. Flavored vinegars and oils are a nice touch, so feel free to experiment with your own combinations.

# Radicchio and Smoked Mozzarella Pasta Salad

*Recently, I served this salad at a garden party for fifty people. The salad dressing is easy to increase; use two parts oil to one part vinegar. For example, for every cup of oil, use ½ cup balsamic vinegar, 8 small shallots, 2 teaspoons salt, and 1 teaspoon black pepper.*

*Dressing:*

2 tablespoons olive oil
1 tablespoon balsamic vinegar
1 small shallot, minced
¼ teaspoon salt
⅛ teaspoon freshly ground
  pepper

*Salad:*

6 ounces farfalle pasta
1 medium fennel bulb, trimmed
  and cut into thin strips (2 cups)
1 cup shredded radicchio
4 ounces smoked mozzarella,
  coarsely grated
2 tablespoons slivered fresh
  basil, for garnish

1. Whisk all of the dressing ingredients together with 1 tablespoon water in a 1-cup measure.

2. Cook the pasta according to the package directions, drain, and cool slightly. Combine the pasta with the fennel, radicchio, and mozzarella in a large bowl. Whisk the dressing, pour over the salad, and toss. Garnish with the basil. Serve at room temperature or chilled.

SERVES 4

Kilocalories 311 Kc • Protein 14 Gm • Fat 13 Gm • Percent of calories from fat 38% • Cholesterol 57 mg • Dietary Fiber 1 Gm • Sodium 311 mg • Calcium 222 mg

# Frisee with Hazelnut Oil and Roquefort

*Frisee, also, known as curly endive, is the young shoot of endive (not to be confused with Belgian endive). It is less bitter and more tender than fully grown endive and has delicate small, frizzy leaves.*

4 cups frisee
¼ cup crumbled Roquefort cheese

1 tablespoon red wine vinegar
¼ teaspoon salt
¼ teaspoon freshly ground pepper

*Dressing:*

1 tablespoon French hazelnut oil

1. Combine the frisee and cheese in a serving bowl.
2. Whisk all the dressing ingredients together with 1 tablespoon water in a 1-cup measure. Drizzle over the salad mixture, toss, and serve.

SERVES 4

**Variation:** Substitute 5 cups mesclun for the frisee, ¼ cup Gorgonzola cheese for the Roquefort, and use walnut oil instead of hazelnut oil. Follow the same instructions.

Kilocalories 92 Kc • Protein 4 Gm • Fat 8 Gm • Percent of calories from fat 75% • Cholesterol 13 mg • Dietary Fiber 2 Gm • Sodium 413 mg • Calcium 121 mg

# Tropical Spinach Salad

6 cups chopped spinach
½ cup thinly sliced red onion

*Dressing:*

1 can (8 ounces) crushed
    pineapple in natural juice
½ small banana
1 tablespoon raspberry vinegar

1 tablespoon honey
½ teaspoon salt
¼ teaspoon freshly ground
    pepper
⅛ teaspoon ground allspice
1 tablespoon chopped
    macadamia nuts

1. Place the spinach on a serving platter; top with the onion.

2. Combine all of the dressing ingredients, except the nuts, with 2 tablespoons water in a blender and process until smooth. Drizzle the dressing over the salad, toss and sprinkle with the nuts. Serve immediately.

SERVES 4

Kilocalories 89 Kc • Protein 3 Gm • Fat 2 Gm • Percent of calories from fat 18% • Cholesterol 0 mg • Dietary Fiber 4 Gm • Sodium 359 mg • Calcium 99 mg

# Spicy Pink Bean Salad

*Pink beans are also known as* habichuelas rosas *and are available in the specialty food section of supermarkets.*

1 bunch arugula, trimmed and
   cut into thin strips
1 bunch beet greens, trimmed
   and chopped
1 can (15 ounces) pink beans,
   rinsed and drained
¼ cup chopped onion

*Dressing:*

2 tablespoons balsamic vinegar
2 tablespoons hot pepper oil*
½ teaspoon salt

   1. Combine the greens on a serving platter. Top with the beans and onion.

   2. Whisk all of the dressing ingredients together in a 1-cup measure; drizzle over the salad and serve.

SERVES 6

*Hot pepper oil is sold at specialty food stores. To make your own, combine 2 tablespoons olive oil, and ¼ teaspoon cayenne pepper. Add more pepper to taste for a spicier oil.

**Variation:** Use any leftover salad for a burrito. Place the leftovers in a nonstick skillet and cook, covered, over medium heat for 2 minutes, stirring once. Place on a tortilla and top with salsa and shredded low-fat cheese. Roll and serve with a knife and fork.

Kilocalories 191Kc • Protein 10 Gm • Fat 5 Gm • Percent of calories from fat 23% • Cholesterol 0 mg • Dietary Fiber 7 Gm • Sodium 485 mg • Calcium 214 mg

# Taco Salad

*This salad is easier to make than it appears because both the dressing and the salad shells may be made ahead.*

*Dressing:*

¾ cup nonfat buttermilk
½ avocado, peeled and
  chopped
1 small onion, halved
1 canned green chili pepper,
  drained
½ teaspoon salt

*Salad:*

12 (6-inch) corn tortillas
3 cups shredded iceberg lettuce
2 cups cooked kidney beans
1 cup chopped fresh tomato
1 cup shredded Monterey Jack
  cheese (about 4 ounces)
¼ cup sliced scallions

1. Combine all of the dressing ingredients in a blender and puree until smooth. Refrigerate until ready to use.

2. Preheat the oven to 400°. Place 1 tortilla in each of 6 custard cups, gently pushing it down to fit. Place the cups on a baking sheet and bake 5 minutes; cool. Remove the shells from the cups and repeat with the remaining tortillas until all are baked.

3. To prepare the salad, combine the lettuce, beans, tomato, cheese, and scallions. Fill each tortilla cup with about ¾ cup of the bean mixture. Spoon 2 tablespoons of the dressing over each. Place 2 tortilla cups on each of 6 plates and serve.

SERVES 6

Kilocalories 307Kc • Protein 14 Gm • Fat 11 Gm • Percent of calories from fat 29% • Cholesterol 21 mg • Dietary Fiber 9 Gm • Sodium 740 mg • Calcium 296 mg

# Mixed Salad with Parmesan Curls

*Dressing:*

2 tablespoons chicken broth
1 tablespoon extra-virgin olive oil
1 tablespoon balsamic vinegar
¼ teaspoon salt

*Salad:*

6 ripe plum tomatoes (or 3 medium regular tomatoes), thinly sliced lengthwise

2 bunches arugula, trimmed and coarsely chopped
3 thin slices red onion, separated into rings

*Garnish:*

⅓ cup (about 1 ounce) Parmesan cheese curls made with a swivel-blade peeler

1. Whisk all of the dressing ingredients together in a 1-cup measure.

2. Arrange the tomatoes around a serving platter; top with arugula and onion. Drizzle with dressing and garnish with Parmesan curls. Serve immediately.

SERVES 4

**Variation:** Dressing: Substitute 2 tablespoons orange juice for the chicken broth and add freshly ground pepper to taste. Salad: Substitute peeled orange sections for the tomatoes; eliminate the cheese.

**Kilocalories 110 Kc • Protein 6 Gm • Fat 6 Gm • Percent of calories from fat 49% • Cholesterol 6 mg • Dietary Fiber 1 Gm • Sodium 311 mg • Calcium 234 mg**

# Sicilian Grilled Swordfish Salad

1¼ pounds swordfish steak
(about 1 inch thick)

*Marinade:*

⅓ cup fresh orange juice
2 tablespoons chopped red
onion

1½ tablespoons olive oil
1 tablespoon fresh rosemary
(1 teaspoon dried)
2 teaspoons capers
¼ teaspoon red pepper flakes

4 cups bitter greens (arugula,
dandelion, chicory, mizuna)

1. Rinse the fish and pat it dry with paper towels; set aside.

2. To prepare the marinade, whisk the juice, onion, oil, rosemary, capers, and pepper flakes together in a shallow bowl. Add the fish; turn to coat. Cover and refrigerate up to 3 hours, turning occasionally. Drain and add the marinade to a small saucepan.

3. Coat a grill or broiler rack with vegetable oil spray. Preheat the grill or broiler. Grill or broil the fish 4 inches from the hot coals (heat), 4 to 5 minutes on each side.

4. Meanwhile, bring the marinade to a boil over medium heat. Remove it from the heat and keep it warm.

5. Cut the fish into 2-inch chunks. Combine with the greens in a serving bowl. Drizzle with the marinade, toss, and serve.

SERVES 4

Kilocalories 248 Kc • Protein 30 Gm • Fat 11 Gm • Percent of calories from fat 41%
• Cholesterol 55 mg • Dietary Fiber 2 Gm • Sodium 214 mg • Calcium 98 mg

# Greek Salad with Chickpeas

*This is a good lunch-size salad.*

*Dressing:*

4 teaspoons olive oil
1 tablespoon fresh lemon juice
1 teaspoon red wine vinegar
1 teaspoon dried oregano
½ teaspoon salt
¼ teaspoon freshly ground
   pepper

*Salad:*

1 cup cooked chickpeas
2 medium tomatoes, quartered
   and thinly sliced
½ cup chopped red onion
2 ounces basil and tomato-
   flavored feta cheese, crumbled
3 cups chopped fresh spinach
8 oil-cured black olives, optional

1. Whisk all of the dressing ingredients together in a 1-cup measure with 1 tablespoon water.

2. Combine the chickpeas, tomatoes, onion, and cheese in a medium bowl. Toss with half the dressing. Arrange the spinach on a serving platter, top with the salad, drizzle with the remaining dressing, and serve with the olives, if desired.

SERVES 4

Kilocalories 172 Kc • Protein 7 Gm • Fat 9 Gm • Percent of calories from fat 45%
• Cholesterol 13 mg • Dietary Fiber 5 Gm • Sodium 743 mg • Calcium 151 mg

# Cucumber and Watercress Salad

1 large seedless cucumber, pared
    and sliced (about 4 cups)
1 bunch watercress, trimmed and
    chopped (about 3 cups)
¼ cup chopped onion

*Dressing:*

¼ cup nonfat sour cream or light
    mayonnaise
¼ cup 1% milk
2 tablespoons tarragon vinegar
2 teaspoons sugar
½ teaspoon dry mustard
¼ teaspoon salt
2 tablespoons chopped fresh
    tarragon for garnish, optional

1. Combine the cucumber, watercress, and onion in a serving bowl.

2. Whisk all of the dressing ingredients together in a 1-cup measure.
Pour over the salad and toss. Garnish with tarragon, if desired.

SERVES 6

Kilocalories 33 Kc • Protein 2 Gm • Fat 0 Gm • Percent of calories from fat 5%
• Cholesterol 0 mg • Dietary Fiber 1 Gm • Sodium 121 mg • Calcium 55 mg

# Fig and Blood Orange Salad

*Blood oranges, a sweet variety with garnet-colored flesh, are very popular in Sicily and other parts of Europe. Their rind, orange with large splotches of scarlet, makes them quite distinctive. They are now grown in the United States and often can be found at the local supermarket.*

*Salad:*

- 3 blood oranges (or other seedless orange), peeled, thinly sliced, and coarsely chopped
- 3 cups chopped red leaf lettuce
- 2 cups chopped red oak (leaf) lettuce
- 1 cup chopped escarole hearts (tender interior of escarole)
- 12 ripe purple figs, cut in quarters

*Dressing:*

- ¼ cup fresh orange juice
- 2 tablespoons white wine vinegar
- 2 tablespoons olive oil
- 1 tablespoon honey
- ½ teaspoon grated orange zest
- ¼ teaspoon salt
- ¼ teaspoon freshly ground pepper
- Slivered Parmesan or Asiago cheese for garnish, optional

1. Combine all of the salad ingredients in a serving bowl.

2. Whisk all of the dressing ingredients with 2 tablespoons water in a 1-cup measure; pour over the salad and toss. Garnish with cheese, if desired. Serve immediately.

SERVES 6

Kilocalories 183 Kc • Protein 2 Gm • Fat 5 Gm • Percent of calories from fat 23% • Cholesterol 0 mg • Dietary Fiber 4 Gm • Sodium 7 mg • Calcium 108 mg

# Holiday Salad with Cranberry Sauce Dressing

*Festive, fruity, and fun.*

6 cups (packed) chopped fresh
  spinach
2 cups chopped radicchio

½ cup plain nonfat yogurt
2 tablespoons raspberry vinegar
⅛ teaspoon salt
2 tablespoons chopped walnuts

*Dressing:*

½ cup whole-berry cranberry
  sauce (preferably homemade)

1. Place the spinach and radicchio in a large serving bowl.

2. To prepare the dressing, whisk the cranberry sauce, yogurt, vinegar, and salt in a 2-cup measure. Drizzle over the salad mixture and toss. Sprinkle with the walnuts and serve.

SERVES 6

Kilocalories 78 Kc • Protein 3 Gm • Fat 2 Gm • Percent of calories from fat 20%
• Cholesterol 0 mg • Dietary Fiber 2 Gm • Sodium 117 mg • Calcium 99 mg

# Mesclun with Hazelnut Cream Dressing

*I always have one or two nut oils in my pantry. They make great-tasting dressings.*

8 cups mesclun

*Dressing:*

2 tablespoons heavy cream
1 tablespoon champagne vinegar
2 teaspoons hazelnut oil

1 to 2 tablespoons 1% milk
1 small shallot, minced
1 teaspoon chopped fresh
  rosemary (¼ teaspoon dried)
¼ teaspoon salt
2 tablespoons chopped, skinned,
  toasted hazelnuts

1. Place the mesclun in a large serving bowl.

2. To prepare the dressing, whisk the cream, vinegar, and oil together in a 1-cup measure (the mixture will get very thick). Whisk the 1 tablespoon milk into the mixture to thin it (if you prefer a thinner dressing, add the additional tablespoon of milk); add the shallot, rosemary, and salt. Drizzle the dressing over the salad mixture and toss. Sprinkle with the nuts and serve.

SERVES 4

Kilocalories 95 Kc • Protein 2 Gm • Fat 8 Gm • Percent of calories from fat 74%
• Cholesterol 10 mg • Dietary Fiber 1 Gm • Sodium 197 mg • Calcium 78 mg

# Fruit and Cabbage Slaw

*This sweet and sour slaw is an easy way to satisfy the new food pyramid's suggestion to eat five ½-cup servings of fruits and vegetables a day.*

3 cups shredded red cabbage
3 Golden Delicious apples, cored
  and chopped
1 can (8 ounces) crushed
  pineapple in natural juice,
  undrained
⅓ cup dried cherries or
  raisins

¼ cup fresh lemon juice
2 teaspoons sugar
1 tablespoon chopped fresh mint
  (1 teaspoon dried)
½ teaspoon salt
¼ teaspoon freshly ground
  pepper

1. Combine the cabbage, apples, pineapple, and cherries in a serving bowl.

2. Whisk the lemon juice, sugar, mint, salt, and pepper together in a 1-cup measure. Pour over the mixture in the bowl. Cover and refrigerate (up to 2 hours), tossing occasionally until ready to serve.

SERVES 4

Kilocalories 151 Kc • Protein 2 Gm • Fat 1 Gm • Percent of calories from fat 3%
• Cholesterol 0 mg • Dietary Fiber 4 Gm • Sodium 299 mg • Calcium 48 mg

# Red Boston and Chicory Salad with Macadamia Oil

*This is what I call the "tough but tender" salad. Boston lettuce has soft, delicate leaves while chicory has curly and robust leaves, adding texture and contrast. Although the recipe calls for macadamia nut oil, which is quite distinctive and delicious, any other nut oil in your pantry would be suitable.*

3 cups chopped red Boston lettuce (or green if the red variety is unavailable)
3 cups chopped chicory
1 Red Delicious apple (or other red-skinned apple), cored and chopped

2 teaspoons fresh lemon juice

*Dressing:*

1½ tablespoons macadamia oil
1 tablespoon fresh lemon juice
¼ teaspoon salt

1. Place the greens in a serving bowl. Combine the apple and lemon juice in a small bowl. Add to the greens.

2. Whisk all of the dressing ingredients together with 1 tablespoon water in a 1-cup measure. Drizzle over the salad mixture and toss. Serve immediately.

SERVES 4

Kilocalories 79 Kc • Protein 3 Gm • Fat 3 Gm • Percent of calories from fat 29% • Cholesterol 0 mg • Dietary Fiber 6 Gm • Sodium 209 mg • Calcium 151 mg

# Radicchio Cups with Wild Mushroom Salad

*This recipe may be halved.*

*Dressing:*

2 tablespoons hazelnut oil
1 tablespoon sherry vinegar
1 small garlic clove, minced
1 tablespoon chopped fresh dill
   (1 teaspoon dried)
½ teaspoon salt
¼ teaspoon freshly ground
   pepper

*Salad:*

4 cups fresh wild mushrooms
   (oyster, chanterelles, shiitake,
   porcini), cleaned and cut into
   strips (if using shiitake, discard
   stems)
½ cup chopped fresh flat-leaf
   parsley
8 large radicchio lettuce leaves

1. Whisk all of the dressing ingredients together with ½ cup water in a medium bowl. Add the mushrooms and parsley; toss to coat. Cover with plastic wrap and refrigerate up to 4 hours, stirring occasionally.

2. Place the radicchio leaves on salad plates and fill with the mushroom salad. Serve immediately.

SERVES 8

Kilocalories 52 Kc • Protein 1 Gm • Fat 4 Gm • Percent of calories from fat 57% • Cholesterol 0 mg • Dietary Fiber 1 Gm • Sodium 151 mg • Calcium 10 mg

# Hearts of Palm and Watercress Salad

*If you don't have fresh tarragon, I suggest using tarragon vinegar instead of red wine vinegar.*

*Dressing:*

**2 tablespoons red wine vinegar**
**1½ tablespoons olive oil**
**2 teaspoons finely chopped fresh tarragon**
**½ teaspoon Dijon mustard**
**¼ teaspoon salt**

*Salad:*

**Boston or Bibb lettuce leaves (to line plates)**

**2 cups drained canned hearts of palm, sliced diagonally into 1-inch pieces**
**1 bunch watercress, trimmed and coarsely chopped (about 3 cups)**

*Garnish:*

**¼ cup finely diced red bell pepper**
**¼ cup finely diced zucchini**

1. Whisk all of the dressing ingredients together with 1 tablespoon water in a 1-cup measure.

2. Arrange the lettuce on 4 salad plates. Combine the hearts of palm and watercress in a medium bowl. Spoon equal amounts onto the lettuce. Drizzle with the dressing and garnish with the pepper and zucchini. Serve immediately.

SERVES 4

Kilocalories 62 Kc • Protein 2 Gm • Fat 5 Gm • Percent of calories from fat 72% • Cholesterol 0 mg • Dietary Fiber 2 Gm • Sodium 164 mg • Calcium 38 mg

# Plantain and Red Leaf Salad

*Plantains are ripe when the skin turns black, they yield slightly to the touch, and the inside is a light coral color.*

1 large ripe plantain, sliced
6 cups red leaf lettuce

1 tablespoon walnut oil
1 teaspoon sugar
¼ teaspoon salt

*Dressing:*

2 tablespoons apple cider
   vinegar

1. Preheat the oven to 400°. Coat a baking pan with vegetable oil spray. Arrange the plantain in a single layer in the pan. Bake 10 minutes. Turn the slices and bake 10 minutes longer. Remove from the pan and cool.

2. Place the lettuce in a serving bowl. Add the plantains.

3. Whisk all of the dressing ingredients together with 2 tablespoons water in a 1-cup measure. Drizzle over the salad mixture and toss.

SERVES 4

Kilocalories 105 Kc • Protein 2 Gm • Fat 4 Gm • Percent of calories from fat 29% • Cholesterol 0 mg • Dietary Fiber 3 Gm • Sodium 155 mg • Calcium 58 mg

# Romaine and Red Pepper Salad with Herbed Cheese Dressing

6 cups chopped romaine lettuce
1 cup julienne of red pepper
¼ cup minced onion

1 tablespoon chopped fresh flat-leaf parsley
¼ teaspoon spicy salt-free seasoning

*Dressing:*

½ cup nonfat cottage cheese
3 tablespoons skim milk

1. Combine the lettuce, pepper, and onion in a serving bowl.

2. Place the dressing ingredients in a blender or a small food processor and process for a few seconds until smooth. Drizzle over the salad and toss. Serve immediately.

SERVES 4

Kilocalories 57 Kc • Protein 6 Gm • Fat 0 Gm • Percent of calories from fat 5% • Cholesterol 3 mg • Dietary Fiber 3 Gm • Sodium 108 mg • Calcium 68 mg

# Red Belgian Endive with Creamy Egg Dressing

*The more common pale green Belgian endive may be substituted.*

3 medium heads red Belgian endive

*Dressing:*

2 large hard-cooked eggs, quartered
2 tablespoons 1% milk

1 tablespoon walnut oil
2 teaspoons red wine vinegar
¼ teaspoon salt
⅛ teaspoon freshly ground pepper
1 tablespoon chopped fresh flat-leaf parsley, for garnish

1. Slice, then chop 1 head of endive. Place in a small bowl.

2. Combine all of the dressing ingredients, except the parsley, in a small food processor. Process until smooth and creamy. Pour over the endive and toss.

3. Separate the leaves from the remaining heads of endive. Line 4 salad plates with endive leaves in a spoke fashion. Spoon the salad onto the center of each plate and sprinkle with the parsley. Serve immediately.

SERVES 4

Kilocalories 84 Kc • Protein 4 Gm • Fat 6 Gm • Percent of calories from fat 65% • Cholesterol 106 mg • Dietary Fiber 2 Gm • Sodium 182 mg • Calcium 35 mg

# Middle Eastern Cabbage Salad

*Tahini, a thick sesame paste, often goes unused because it settles to the bottom of the can and becomes as hard as a brick. To solve this problem, first pour the oil into a blender container, then dig out the hardened paste from the can with a knife or fork and add to the blender. Puree and pour back into the can. Refrigerate and the paste will remain blended. If you rarely use tahini, a great substitute that every American household seems to have is peanut butter.*

*Orange-Tahini Dressing:*

3 tablespoons fresh orange juice
2 tablespoons tahini
1 tablespoon reduced-sodium
 soy sauce

*Salad:*

4 cups shredded Chinese or napa
 cabbage
2 cups shredded carrot
1 cup snow peas (about 3
 ounces)
½ cup sliced scallions

1. Whisk the orange juice, tahini, and soy sauce together in a 1-cup measure.

2. Combine the cabbage, carrots, snow peas, and scallions in a serving bowl. Drizzle with the dressing and toss to coat. Serve immediately.

SERVES 6

Kilocalories 80 Kc • Protein 3 Gm • Fat 3 Gm • Percent of calories from fat 37% • Cholesterol 0 mg • Dietary Fiber 2 Gm • Sodium 134 mg • Calcium 71 mg

# Beet Greens and Butterhead Lettuce with Buttermilk Dressing

*An interesting play on texture, color, and taste.*

*Dressing:*

¼ cup nonfat buttermilk
1 tablespoon red wine vinegar
1 garlic clove, crushed
½ teaspoon crumbled dried
  tarragon
¼ teaspoon salt

¼ teaspoon black pepper, very
  coarsely ground

*Salad:*

3 cups chiffonade of beet greens
3 cups torn butterhead or Boston
  lettuce

1. Whisk all of the dressing ingredients together in a 1-cup measure; let it stand for 30 minutes. Discard the garlic.

2. Place the beet greens and lettuce in a serving bowl. Drizzle the dressing over the salad mixture, toss, and serve.

SERVES 4

Kilocalories 33 Kc • Protein 3 Gm • Fat 0 Gm • Percent of calories from fat 9% • Cholesterol 1 mg • Dietary Fiber 2 Gm • Sodium 322 mg • Calcium 110 mg

# Green Bean, Tomato, and Field Green Salad

*This low-fat salad may be made ahead and refrigerated except for the field greens. Add those just before serving.*

12 ounces green beans, trimmed and cut in half (or one 10-ounce package frozen cut green beans, cooked and drained)

*Spinach-Parsley Dressing:*

1 cup (packed) chopped fresh spinach
½ cup chopped fresh flat-leaf parsley

⅓ cup chicken broth
2 tablespoons fresh lemon juice
2 tablespoons chopped red onion
1 small garlic clove
Salt and freshly ground pepper

2 medium ripe tomatoes, cut into 8 wedges
2 cups field greens

1. Place the green beans in a collapsible steamer basket set over simmering water in a wide saucepan. Cover and steam about 10 minutes depending on your desired doneness. Cool and dry with paper towels. Place in a serving bowl and refrigerate 30 minutes.

2. Combine all of the dressing ingredients in a blender or food processor. Puree until smooth. Add salt and pepper to taste.

3. Add the tomatoes and greens to the chilled green beans. Pour the dressing over the salad, toss, and serve immediately.

SERVES 4

Kilocalories 69 Kc • Protein 4 Gm • Fat 1 Gm • Percent of calories from fat 10% • Cholesterol 0 mg • Dietary Fiber 5 Gm • Sodium 52 mg • Calcium 121 mg

# Mom's Chicory Salad

*Mom served salad at lunch and dinner, seven days a week. The lettuce of choice was iceberg, dressed with oil, red wine vinegar, and lots of salt. Occasionally, she'd sneak in the following chicory salad. We all complained. Now, I'm grateful.*

**6 cups chopped chicory**

*Dressing:*

**3 tablespoons fresh lemon juice**
**1 tablespoon olive oil**

**½ teaspoon salt**
**¼ teaspoon freshly ground pepper**

1. Place the chicory in a serving bowl.
2. Whisk all of the dressing ingredients together with 1 tablespoon water in a 1-cup measure. Drizzle over the chicory, toss, and serve.

SERVES 4

Kilocalories 95 Kc • Protein 5 Gm • Fat 4 Gm • Percent of calories from fat 34% • Cholesterol 0 mg • Dietary Fiber 11 Gm • Sodium 412 mg • Calcium 272 mg

# Baby Kohlrabi and Greens Salad with Warm Cranberry-Vinegar Dressing

*Kohlrabi bulbs are very tender when steamed. The leaves are slightly leathery but full of flavor.*

2 bunches (about 12 ounces) baby kohlrabi with leaves

1 tablespoon honey
1 tablespoon olive oil
½ teaspoon kosher salt

*Dressing:*

1 tablespoon cranberry vinegar (or other slightly sweet vinegar)

1. Rinse the kohlrabi, cut off its leaves, and place the leaves in cold water. Cut the kohlrabi bulbs into ½-inch cubes and place in a collapsible steamer basket set over simmering water in a wide saucepan. Cover and steam until tender, about 12 minutes. Carefully lift the basket from the saucepan with a long-handled fork and place it in the sink to cool.

2. Place all of the dressing ingredients in a small saucepan over medium heat. Bring to a boil, stirring to dissolve the honey. Remove from the heat and keep warm.

3. Drain the kohlrabi leaves and spin dry. Chop them coarsely and place them in a serving bowl with the steamed kohlrabi. Drizzle the dressing over the mixture, toss, and serve.

SERVES 6

Kilocalories 40 Kc • Protein 1 Gm • Fat 2 Gm • Percent of calories from fat 48% • Cholesterol 0 mg • Dietary Fiber 1 Gm • Sodium 200 mg • Calcium 8 mg

# Swiss Cheese, "Bacon," and Spinach Salad

*Dressing:*

2 tablespoons fresh lemon juice
1½ tablespoons vegetable oil
1 teaspoon grainy mustard
½ teaspoon salt
¼ teaspoon freshly ground
    pepper
4 ounces small fresh mushrooms,
    trimmed and sliced

*Salad:*

1 package (10 ounces) fresh
    spinach, trimmed and chopped
4 ounces low-fat Swiss
    cheese, cut into julienne
    strips
5 strips cooked turkey bacon or
    meatless bacon,
    crumbled

1. Combine all of the dressing ingredients, except the mushrooms, with 2½ tablespoons water in a serving bowl. Add the mushrooms and let the mixture stand for 30 minutes.

2. Add the spinach to the mushroom mixture and toss to coat. Top with the cheese and bacon and serve.

SERVES 4

Kilocalories 206 Kc • Protein 18 Gm • Fat 14 Gm • Percent of calories from fat 54%
• Cholesterol 38 mg • Dietary Fiber 2 Gm • Sodium 724 mg • Calcium 350 mg

# Roasted Chicken and Spinach Salad in Honey Mustard Vinaigrette

*This is a delicious way to use leftover chicken in a main-course dish.*

1 package (10 ounces) fresh
   spinach, trimmed and chopped
2 cups cubed roasted chicken
   pieces
3 tablespoons minced fresh
   chives or scallions

*Dressing:*

2 tablespoons honey mustard
1½ tablespoons olive oil
2 teaspoons apple cider vinegar
¼ teaspoon salt
¼ teaspoon freshly ground
   pepper

1. Combine the spinach, chicken, and chives in a serving bowl.

2. Whisk all of the dressing ingredients together with 3 tablespoons water in a 1-cup measure. Drizzle over the salad mixture, toss, and serve.

SERVES 4

Kilocalories 206 Kc • Protein 24 Gm • Fat 9 Gm • Percent of calories from fat 39% • Cholesterol 60 mg • Dietary Fiber 2 Gm • Sodium 350 mg • Calcium 90 mg

# Italian Tomato Salad with Arugula

*For the best flavor, use ripe tomatoes in season.*

3 cups coarsely chopped
    tomatoes (about 1¼ pounds)
⅓ cup chopped red onion
1 tablespoon extra-virgin olive oil
2 tablespoons red wine vinegar

2 teaspoons dried oregano
½ teaspoon salt
Freshly ground pepper
2 cups (packed) chopped arugula

1. Combine all of the ingredients, except the arugula, in a serving bowl; let the mixture stand at room temperature for 1 to 2 hours. (The salad may be refrigerated overnight; bring to room temperature before serving.)

2. To serve, add the arugula to the tomato mixture, toss, and serve.

SERVES 6

Kilocalories 48 Kc • Protein 1 Gm • Fat 3 Gm • Percent of calories from fat 47% • Cholesterol 0 mg • Dietary Fiber 1 Gm • Sodium 205 mg • Calcium 26 mg

# Smoked Chicken Salad with Field Greens

*Vinaigrette:*

2 tablespoons extra-virgin olive oil
2 tablespoons balsamic vinegar
1 teaspoon grated orange zest
¼ teaspoon salt
¼ teaspoon freshly ground pepper

*Salad:*

8 ounces smoked chicken (or turkey), cut in julienne strips
1 cup chopped jicama
½ cup small red seedless grapes
½ cup small green seedless grapes
¼ cup sliced almonds
4 cups field greens (arugula, mache, frisee, dandelion)

1. Whisk all of the vinaigrette ingredients together with 2 tablespoons water in a 1-cup measure.

2. To prepare the salad, combine the chicken, jicama, grapes, and almonds in a serving bowl. Pour the vinaigrette over the salad, and toss.

3. Garnish 4 plates with the wild greens; spoon the salad onto each plate and serve.

SERVES 4

Kilocalories 249 Kc • Protein 17 Gm • Fat 15 Gm • Percent of calories from fat 52% • Cholesterol 30 mg • Dietary Fiber 7 Gm • Sodium 723 mg • Calcium 154 mg

# Asian Tofu Salad

*If tofu mayonnaise is unavailable, use light mayonnaise.*

*Salad:*

1 package (14 ounces) firm tofu, drained and patted dry with paper towels, cut into bite-size cubes

2 cups thinly sliced bok choy, green part only

1 medium red bell pepper, seeded and cut into thin strips

½ cup fresh bean sprouts, rinsed and chopped

½ cup drained canned bamboo shoots

*Dressing:*

¼ cup reduced-sodium soy sauce

¼ cup sliced scallions

3 tablespoons tofu mayonnaise

1 tablespoon rice vinegar

1 teaspoon chili paste

1. Combine all of the salad ingredients in a serving bowl.

2. Whisk all of the dressing ingredients together in a 1-cup measure. Pour over the salad, toss, and serve.

SERVES 4

Kilocalories 173 Kc • Protein 12 Gm • Fat 11 Gm • Percent of calories from fat 55% • Cholesterol 6 mg • Dietary Fiber 2 Gm • Sodium 753 mg • Calcium 102 mg

# Belgian Endive and Scallop Salad with Roasted Red Pepper Dressing

1 cup chicken or fish broth
1 pound sea scallops, halved
2 cups blanched broccoli florets
1 medium head Belgian endive,
    trimmed and sliced
16 niçoise olives

*Dressing:*

1 cup roasted red peppers
2 tablespoons olive oil
2 teaspoons red wine vinegar
2 garlic cloves
¼ teaspoon salt
Freshly ground pepper

1. Bring the broth to a boil in a medium saucepan; reduce the heat to medium. Add the scallops and poach for 6 to 8 minutes or until opaque. Drain and dry them thoroughly on paper towels.

2. Combine the scallops, broccoli, endive, and olives in a serving bowl.

3. Puree all of the dressing ingredients in a blender or a small food processor. Pour the dressing over the salad, toss, and serve.

SERVES 4

Kilocalories 219 Kc • Protein 22 Gm • Fat 10 Gm • Percent of calories from fat 42%
• Cholesterol 39 mg • Dietary Fiber 3 Gm • Sodium 518 mg • Calcium 74 mg

# Spinach, Endive, and Strawberry Salad

16 large fresh spinach leaves, rinsed and dried
2 heads Belgian endive, trimmed and leaves separated
3 cups low-fat cottage cheese
1 cup alfalfa sprouts
2 cups whole strawberries, hulled and halved

*Dressing:*

¼ cup fresh orange juice
2 tablespoons vegetable oil
1 teaspoon grated orange zest
⅛ teaspoon ground ginger
Freshly ground pepper

1. Divide the spinach among 4 plates; arrange the endive leaves in a spoke-like pattern on the spinach. Place ¾ cup cottage cheese in the center of each plate; sprinkle evenly with the alfalfa sprouts. Place ½ cup of the strawberries, around the cottage cheese, on the endive leaves on each plate.

2. Combine all of the dressing ingredients with 1 tablespoon water in a 1-cup measure. Drizzle over the salads and serve.

SERVES 4

Kilocalories 226 Kc • Protein 23 Gm • Fat 9 Gm • Percent of calories from fat 35% • Cholesterol 7 mg • Dietary Fiber 3 Gm • Sodium 702 mg • Calcium 142 mg

# Greens with Sun-Dried Tomato Dressing

3 cups chopped chicory
3 cups coarsely chopped arugula
2 cups shredded radicchio

*Dressing:*

2 large sun-dried tomatoes,
   quartered and rehydrated

2 tablespoons extra-virgin olive
   oil
2 teaspoons balsamic vinegar
1 garlic clove
1 teaspoon dried basil
¼ teaspoon salt
½ cup rehydrated sun-dried
   tomatoes cut in julienne strips,
   for garnish (optional)

1. Arrange the greens on a serving platter.

2. Puree all of the dressing ingredients in a blender with ½ cup water. Drizzle over the greens and garnish with the chopped tomatoes, if desired. Serve immediately.

SERVES 6

Kilocalories 73 Kc • Protein 2 Gm • Fat 5 Gm • Percent of calories from fat 55%
• Cholesterol 0 mg • Dietary Fiber 4 Gm • Sodium 190 mg • Calcium 117 mg

# Romaine and Cucumbers in Green Herb Dressing

*Romaine lettuce is easy to cut with scissors. Just cut down the center rib dividing the leaf in two, then stack the cut leaves. Using a scissors again, cut across to the width you want. This method eliminates trying to eat leaves that are 5 inches across with a big knob in the center. This also cuts down on the cleaning bills—no more splattered silk blouses and ties.*

*Green Herb Dressing:*

¼ cup packed fresh flat-leaf parsley
¼ cup plain low-fat yogurt
1 tablespoon fresh tarragon leaves
1 tablespoon vegetable oil
2 teaspoons apple cider vinegar
¼ teaspoon salt
⅛ teaspoon ground coriander

*Salad:*

1 large seedless cucumber, pared and sliced (about 4 cups)
3 cups sliced romaine lettuce
½ cup thinly sliced red onion
3 tablespoons sunflower seeds for garnish, optional

1. Combine all of the dressing ingredients in a blender or a small food processor with 2 tablespoons water and process about 30 seconds until the parsley is chopped.*

2. Combine the cucumber, lettuce, and red onion in a serving bowl. Pour the dressing over the salad, toss, and sprinkle with the sunflower seeds, if desired. Serve immediately.

SERVES 6

*Dressing made in a blender will be greener because the parsley is more finely minced.

**Kilocalories 46 Kc • Protein 2 Gm • Fat 3 Gm • Percent of calories from fat 48% • Cholesterol 1 mg • Dietary Fiber 2 Gm • Sodium 109 mg • Calcium 44 mg**

# Caesar Salad with Parmesan Potato Chips

*Anchovies are salty so I don't think this dressing needs more salt, but your taste buds, like my husband's, may be different from mine. A note to the wary: Egg substitute is pasteurized, so there's no need to worry about this Caesar dressing.*

*Parmesan Potato Chips:*

2 medium baking potatoes (about 10 ounces), washed, scrubbed, and thinly sliced (⅛ inch thick)
¼ cup grated Parmesan cheese
Kosher or coarse salt

*Salad:*

2 garlic cloves, crushed
¼ cup egg substitute

2 tablespoons fresh lemon juice
3 anchovy fillets
1 teaspoon Dijon mustard
1 teaspoon red wine vinegar
1 teaspoon Worcestershire sauce
¼ teaspoon freshly ground pepper
¼ cup extra-virgin olive oil
Salt
1 medium head romaine lettuce, trimmed and cut into bite-size pieces

1. Preheat the oven to 450°.

2. To prepare the Parmesan potato chips, place the sliced potatoes on a baking sheet coated with vegetable oil spray. Sprinkle with the cheese and a little kosher salt (this adds a little texture and makes the potato taste more like a chip.) Bake 12 to 15 minutes until browned and crisp. Cool and remove the chips with a spatula.

3. To prepare the dressing, combine the garlic, egg substitute, lemon juice, anchovies, mustard, vinegar, Worcestershire sauce, and pepper in a blender container and puree. Remove the center of the lid, and with the machine running slowly, add the oil in a thin stream. Season with salt to taste. Pour into a serving bowl. Add the romaine and toss to coat. Serve with the Parmesan potato chips and additional Parmesan, if desired.

SERVES 6

Kilocalories 150 Kc • Protein 4 Gm • Fat 11 Gm • Percent of calories from fat 63%
• Cholesterol 4 mg • Dietary Fiber 1 Gm • Sodium 170 mg • Calcium 64 mg

# Potato Salad on Romaine with Peanut Butter Dressing

*This is a delicious main-dish salad and a great way to use America's favorite food, peanut butter.*

1½ pounds potatoes, pared and cubed
½ teaspoon salt
8 romaine lettuce leaves
3 medium tomatoes, sliced (about 6 cups)
1 cup thinly sliced red onion
1 cup halved fresh mushrooms
¼ cup chopped fresh basil

*Dressing:*

¼ cup smooth peanut butter
½ cup skim milk
2 tablespoons sliced scallions
¼ teaspoon chili powder

1. Place the potatoes in a medium saucepan. Add water to cover and the salt, partially cover, and boil until just tender, about 15 minutes; drain and place in a medium bowl.

2. Arrange the lettuce, tomatoes, onions, and mushrooms around the edge of a large serving platter. Sprinkle with the basil.

3. Whisk all of the dressing ingredients together in a 2-cup measure. Pour half of the dressing over the potatoes and toss. Mound in the center of the vegetables on the platter. Drizzle the remaining dressing over the vegetables.

SERVES 4

Kilocalories 334 Kc • Protein 13 Gm • Fat 10 Gm • Percent of calories from fat 24% • Cholesterol 1 mg • Dietary Fiber 9 Gm • Sodium 429 mg • Calcium 95 mg

# Bibb, Frisee, and Mushrooms in Red Onion Vinaigrette

*Hearts of chicory are a good substitute for frisee.*

3 cups chopped Bibb lettuce
2 cups chopped frisee
1 cup sliced fresh mushrooms

*Dressing:*

½ cup chicken broth or water
½ cup chopped red onion
1 tablespoon balsamic vinegar
2 teaspoons oil
¼ teaspoon salt (a little more if you use water instead of broth)

1. Place the greens and mushrooms in a serving bowl.

2. To prepare the dressing, combine the broth and onion in a small nonstick skillet. Cover and cook over medium heat for 3 minutes. Uncover and cook 1 to 2 minutes longer until almost all of the liquid is absorbed. Remove from the heat and stir in the vinegar, oil, and salt. Pour over the salad mixture and toss. Serve immediately.

SERVES 4

Kilocalories 56 Kc • Protein 2 Gm • Fat 3 Gm • Percent of calories from fat 43%
• Cholesterol 1 mg • Dietary Fiber 2 Gm • Sodium 168 mg • Calcium 44 mg

# Wilted Field Greens with "Bacon" Dressing

6 cups field greens (mesclun or gourmet salad greens)
½ cup sliced scallions
4 radishes, thinly sliced
4 slices turkey bacon or meatless bacon, diced

2 tablespoons fresh lemon juice
2 tablespoons apple cider vinegar
1 teaspoon sugar
1 hard-boiled egg, chopped, for garnish, optional

1. Combine the greens, scallions, and radishes in a serving bowl.

2. Cook the bacon in a medium nonstick skillet over medium heat for 4 minutes or until crisp. Add ¼ cup water, the lemon juice, vinegar, and sugar; cook 2 minutes. Immediately pour over the salad and toss. Garnish with the egg, if desired, and serve.

SERVES 4

Kilocalories 260 Kc • Protein 21 Gm • Fat 5 Gm • Percent of calories from fat 18% • Cholesterol 0 mg • Dietary Fiber 2 Gm • Sodium 1043 mg • Calcium 83 mg

# Arugula and Artichoke Hearts with Blue Cheese Dressing

*This dressing is delicious and may be doubled. Keep a jar of it in the fridge to use on other salads and vegetables.*

2 cups chopped arugula
1 cup quartered cooked
   artichoke hearts
½ cup halved cherry tomatoes

*Dressing:*

¼ cup nonfat buttermilk
¼ cup crumbled blue cheese
¼ teaspoon freshly ground
   pepper

1. Combine the arugula, artichoke hearts, and cherry tomatoes in a serving bowl.

2. Combine all of the dressing ingredients in a blender. Puree until almost smooth (a few lumps of cheese are desirable). Pour over the salad and toss.

SERVES 2

Kilocalories 123 Kc • Protein 8 Gm • Fat 5 Gm • Percent of calories from fat 31%
• Cholesterol 11 mg • Dietary Fiber 5 Gm • Sodium 313 mg • Calcium 185 mg

# Grilled Eggplant and Endive with Roasted Garlic Dressing (Outdoor Grill)

1 medium eggplant (about 1 pound), trimmed and cut into six ½-inch-thick slices*
2 small heads Belgian endive, cut in half lengthwise
2 tablespoons olive oil, optional

*Roasted Garlic Dressing:*

1 bulb garlic
¼ cup vegetable broth or water
2 tablespoons minced fresh basil
1 tablespoon olive oil
¼ teaspoon salt
¼ teaspoon freshly ground pepper

1. Coat the grill rack with vegetable oil spray. Preheat the grill (medium-high heat or medium-hot coals).

2. Place the eggplant in a collapsible steamer basket set over simmering water in a wide saucepan. Cover tightly and steam 5 minutes or until just fork-tender. (This may be done ahead of time.) Pat dry with paper towels. Brush both sides of the eggplant and endive lightly with olive oil or coat with vegetable oil spray and place in a grill basket. Place the basket on the grill and lower the lid. Grill 8 to 10 minutes on each side. The grilled vegetables may stand at room temperature, covered, up to 3 hours.

3. Preheat the oven to 350°.

4. To prepare the dressing, remove the papery skin from the garlic, but keep the bulb intact. Slice off about 1 inch of the garlic top to expose the flesh of each clove; coat the top with vegetable oil spray. Wrap in foil and bake 1 hour until soft and tender.

5. Remove the foil from the garlic and let it cool slightly before separating the cloves. Squeeze the garlic cloves into a 1-cup measure. Whisk with the broth, basil, oil, salt, and pepper until almost smooth. Spoon over the grilled eggplant and endive and serve immediately.

SERVES 6

*There may be leftover eggplant; save for another use.

Kilocalories 52 Kc • Protein 1 Gm • Fat 2 Gm • Percent of calories from fat 39% • Cholesterol 0 mg • Dietary Fiber 3 Gm • Sodium 108 mg • Calcium 25 mg

# Romaine and Radishes in Creamy Garlic Dressing

*Roasted garlic oil is available in specialty food stores. Olive oil may be substituted in this recipe.*

*Creamy Garlic Dressing:*

½ cup part-skim ricotta cheese
2 tablespoons skim milk
1 tablespoon sherry vinegar
1 tablespoon coarsely chopped
    fresh flat-leaf parsley
2 teaspoons roasted garlic oil
1 large garlic clove, cut in half

1 teaspoon Dijon mustard
¼ teaspoon salt

*Salad:*

6 cups chopped romaine lettuce
1 cup chopped radishes

1. Combine all of the dressing ingredients in a food processor or a blender. Process 20 seconds until smooth and creamy.

2. Combine the lettuce and radishes in a serving bowl. Drizzle with the dressing, toss, and serve.

SERVES 4

Kilocalories 75 Kc • Protein 5 Gm • Fat 4 G • Percent of calories from fat 43%
• Cholesterol 0 mg • Dietary Fiber 2 Gm • Sodium 200 mg • Calcium 90 mg

# Bok Choy with Star Anise Dressing

*Star anise is a star-shaped pod native to China. It is similar in flavor to anise seed with a strong licorice taste and is available at most supermarkets.*

*Dressing:*

2 dried star anise pods
2 tablespoons vegetable
  oil
2 tablespoons rice vinegar
¼ teaspoon salt

*Salad:*

4 cups thinly sliced bok choy
1 cup snow peas (about 3 ounces),
  trimmed and cut in half
½ cup sprouted mung beans,
  optional

1. To prepare the dressing, grind the anise pods in a spice grinder or a small food processor. Whisk the ground anise with oil, vinegar, and salt until combined. Cover and refrigerate 2 hours.

2. To prepare the salad, combine the bok choy, snow peas, and mung beans, if desired, in a serving bowl. Whisk the dressing, drizzle over the salad, toss, and serve.

SERVES 4

Kilocalories 86 Kc • Protein 2 Gm • Fat 7 Gm • Percent of calories from fat 74%
• Cholesterol 0 mg • Dietary Fiber 1 Gm • Sodium 157 mg • Calcium 62 mg

# Greens and Grilled Chicken Salad in Warm Ginger Dressing

*Packaged salad greens make this dish a snap.*

¼ cup low-sodium soy sauce
2 tablespoons rice vinegar
2 tablespoons minced fresh ginger
1 tablespoon peanut oil
1 tablespoon (packed) dark
　　brown sugar

12 ounces boneless, skinless thin-
　　sliced chicken breast
1 package (10 ounces) salad
　　mix (iceberg, leaf lettuce,
　　and Chinese cabbage)

1. Whisk the soy sauce, vinegar, gingerroot, oil, and sugar together in a 1-cup measure.

2. Place the chicken in a plastic bowl with a sealable lid. Pour the soy mixture over the chicken. Cover and refrigerate 3 hours or overnight, shaking the bowl occasionally.

3. Remove the chicken from the marinade to a dish. Pour the marinade into a small saucepan and bring to a boil over high heat. Let it boil 1 minute. Remove from the heat, cover, and keep warm.

4. Heat a stovetop ridged grill, coated with vegetable oil spray, over medium heat.

5. Cook the chicken 2 minutes on each side. Cut into thin strips and combine with the salad greens in a large bowl. Pour the warm sauce over the greens and toss. Divide the salad evenly on 3 serving plates. Serve immediately.

SERVES 3

**Variation:** To serve 4, double the marinade. Top each serving of the salad and chicken mixture with ½ cup cooked cellophane noodles; pour the sauce over the mixture and serve immediately.

**Kilocalories 281 Kc • Protein 35 Gm • Fat 9 Gm • Percent of calories from fat 31%
• Cholesterol 86 mg • Dietary Fiber 1 Gm • Sodium 898 mg • Calcium 79 mg**

# Warm Date and Napa Cabbage Salad

*Brett Lewis contributed this award-winning recipe. He is Chef de Cuisine at La Concha Pacific Bistro at The Weston Mission Hills Resort in Rancho Mirage, California.*

4 slices turkey bacon, cut crosswise into ⅛-inch strips
½ cup balsamic vinegar
6 tablespoons fresh orange juice
1 tablespoon date crystals or raw or granulated sugar
2 cups sliced pitted dates (10 ounces)

1 teaspoon grated orange zest
6 cups shredded napa cabbage
1 cup toasted slivered almonds (about 3 ounces)
½ cup julienned carrots
Fried bean thread noodles for garnish, optional

1. Heat a medium nonstick skillet coated with vegetable oil spray over medium heat. Add the bacon and cook about 3 minutes, stirring frequently, until crisp. Stir in the vinegar, juice, and date crystals; add the dates and orange zest and cook 1 minute. Remove from the heat; cover with foil and keep warm.

2. Combine the cabbage, almonds, and carrots in a large bowl. Pour the warm dressing over the mixture and toss. Garnish with fried bean thread noodles, if desired, and serve immediately.

SERVES 6

Kilocalories 300 Kc • Protein 8 Gm • Fat 9 Gm • Percent of calories from fat 23% • Cholesterol 7 mg • Dietary Fiber 9 Gm • Sodium 154 mg • Calcium 100 mg

# 3

# First Courses and Light Meals

Lighter, smaller, healthier, and quicker meals are in vogue and today antipasto is the perfect example of a little meal which illustrates this new trend. Small amounts of roasted or raw vegetables, salads, olives, hearty breads, and a little cheese are often served as the main meal rather than the start of a meal.

First courses, on the other hand, should stimulate the appetite rather than satisfy it. First courses may also double as light lunches. The ubiquitous cold cut sandwiches of the baby boom generation are now second-string choices to more nutritious and exciting foods.

Sautéed greens and roasted vegetables are replacing processed meats as a sandwich ingredient. Focaccia bread with arugula, cheeses, and roasted vegetables and other healthful combinations are popular choices on menus in many restaurants and at specialty food shops. Even the large fast-food chains have joined the bandwagon and now offer alternative choices in prepared sandwiches.

The meals in this chapter are quick and easy to prepare. An added bonus is that these recipes don't require long shopping trips.

# Tofu Salad in Romaine Lettuce

*Tofu-filled rolls are a dieter's delight—vegetarian, no starch, low in fat, and tasty. One of my friends thought the filling tasted just like egg salad. Serve these with rice cakes and fresh fruit to complete this light meal.*

4 ounces firm tofu, drained and
  mashed
½ cup quartered cherry tomatoes
2 tablespoons light mayonnaise
  or tofu mayonnaise

2 teaspoons chopped fresh
  cilantro or a pinch dried
  coriander
¼ teaspoon salt
4 large romaine lettuce leaves*

Combine the tofu, tomatoes, mayonnaise, cilantro, and salt in a small bowl. Trim the lettuce leaves to 8-inch lengths. Place one fourth of the tofu mixture at one end of each leaf and roll, folding in the sides of the leaf (the thick rib will probably snap). Wrap tightly in plastic wrap and refrigerate 2 hours before serving.

SERVES 2

*The salad may also be placed in lettuce cups. In that case use Boston lettuce.

Kilocalories 88 Kc • Protein 5 Gm • Fat 5 Gm • Percent of calories from fat 53% • Cholesterol 0 mg • Dietary Fiber 1 Gm • Sodium 443 mg • Calcium 30 mg

# Turkey Burgers

*These broiled burgers are made with arugula, but any green you like would be suitable as long as it's finely chopped.*

8 ounces ground lean turkey
1 cup (packed) finely chopped arugula
¼ cup bread crumbs
1 tablespoon mustard
1 large egg white
½ teaspoon salt
¼ teaspoon freshly ground pepper
2 hamburger rolls
2 large onion slices for garnish, optional
Arugula leaves for garnish, optional

1. Preheat the broiler

2. Combine the turkey, arugula, bread crumbs, mustard, egg white, salt, and pepper in a medium bowl. Shape the mixture into 2 patties, about 1 inch thick.

3. Place the patties on a rack in a broiler pan. Broil 4 inches from the heat, about 8 minutes on each side or until no longer pink inside. Place each burger on a roll and garnish with the onion and arugula, if desired.

SERVES 2

Kilocalories 392 Kc • Protein 28 Gm • Fat 15 Gm • Percent of calories from fat 35% • Cholesterol 108 mg • Dietary fiber 1 Gm • Sodium 1114 mg • Calcium 149 mg

# Grilled Brie and Watercress on French Bread

4 slices (5 inches long) French bread

1 cup watercress leaves

8 ounces Brie (with rind), thinly sliced

2 tablespoons coarse mustard

1. Slice each length of French bread horizontally. Place one fourth of the watercress and Brie on each bottom slice of bread. Spread the mustard on the top slices and cover to make 4 sandwiches.

2. Coat a stovetop grill with vegetable oil spray. Place over medium heat for 5 minutes. Grill the sandwiches for 2 to 3 minutes on each side, pressing down with a spatula until the cheese melts. Serve immediately.

SERVES 4

**Variation:** Substitute turkey or meatless salami, arugula, and thinly sliced fontina or provolone cheese for an Italian-style sandwich.

Kilocalories 381 Kc • Protein 20 Gm • Fat 17 Gm • Percent of calories from fat 41% • Cholesterol 57 mg • Dietary Fiber 1 Gm • Sodium 870 mg • Calcium 117 mg

# Chicory-Stuffed Yellow Chili Peppers

*This is a very spicy dish. Yellow chili peppers are often packaged and found in the vegetable section of the supermarket.*

¾ cup bran flake cereal
8 yellow chili peppers
1 tablespoon olive oil
4 anchovy fillets, drained and
  rinsed

4 garlic cloves, minced
2½ cups finely chopped chicory
2 cups coarsely chopped chicory,
  for garnish, optional

1. Preheat the oven to 400°. Coat an 8-inch square baking pan with vegetable oil spray.

2. Crush the bran cereal in a sealable plastic bag using a rolling pin.

3. Cut the stems from the peppers by inserting a sharp knife around the base of the stems. Gently pull out the stems and scrape out the seeds; discard.

4. Heat the oil in a small skillet over medium heat. Add the anchovies and mash; cook 1 minute until the anchovies are almost dissolved. Add the garlic and finely chopped chicory, cover, and cook 2 minutes. Stir in the bran and 2 tablespoons of water. Remove from the heat and cool slightly.

5. Stuff each pepper with the chicory mixture and place them in the prepared pan. Bake 10 minutes; turn each pepper over with a spatula or tongs and bake 10 minutes longer. Place some coarsely chopped chicory on each serving plate if desired, and top with 2 stuffed peppers.

SERVES 4

Kilocalories 104 Kc • Protein 5 Gm • Fat 4 Gm • Percent of calories from fat 33% • Cholesterol 3 mg • Dietary Fiber 6 Gm • Sodium 258 mg • Calcium 129 mg

# Cornmeal Wedges with Sautéed Spinach

*To make this recipe less daunting, cook the cornmeal the day before you plan to serve this dish.*

1 cup yellow cornmeal
1½ teaspoons salt
2 tablespoons olive oil
2 garlic cloves, mashed
¼ teaspoon red pepper flakes

1 package (10 ounces) fresh
    spinach, trimmed and chopped
1 tablespoon grated Parmesan
    cheese, optional

1. Whisk the cornmeal and 1 teaspoon salt together with 3 cups cold water in a double boiler over simmering water. Cook, stirring frequently until thickened and creamy, about 15 minutes. Reduce the heat, cover, and cook 20 to 30 minutes longer, stirring occasionally, until very thick and not gritty to the taste.

2. Spoon the cornmeal into an 8-inch square pan coated with vegetable oil spray; spread with a spatula to smooth. Cool and refrigerate, covered, at least 30 minutes.

3. Meanwhile, heat the oil in a large nonstick skillet over high heat. Add the garlic and red pepper; cook 30 seconds until the garlic is lightly browned. Add the spinach and cook 30 seconds, stirring until the spinach is bright green.

4. Reduce the heat, add the remaining ½ teaspoon salt, cover, and cook 3 minutes, stirring once. Keep warm.

5. Preheat the broiler.

6. Invert the cornmeal onto a cutting board and cut into 4 squares. Cut each square into 2 triangles (making 8). Using a spatula, carefully place the wedges on broiler rack coated with vegetable oil spray. Sprinkle with the cheese, if desired. Place the pan 2 inches from the heat and broil for 3 to 4 minutes, or until lightly browned.

7. Place 4 cornmeal wedges in a circle on each plate. Spoon the warm spinach into the center and serve immediately.

SERVES 2

**Variation:** Sautéed Ginger Spinach: Eliminate the red pepper flakes and substitute 1 tablespoon slivered fresh ginger. Also eliminate the Parmesan cheese and sprinkle the cornmeal wedges with a little ground mace before broiling.

Kilocalories 376 Kc • Protein 9 Gm • Fat 16 Gm • Percent of calories from fat 37% • Cholesterol 0 mg • Dietary Fiber 8 Gm • Sodium 1876 mg • Calcium 149 mg

# Collard Greens Tortilla

*The tortilla is the Spanish version of the Italian frittata—basically an egg and vegetable omelet that isn't folded or filled.*

4 large eggs
2 egg whites
1 package (10 ounces) chopped
 frozen collard greens, thawed,
 drained, and squeezed
½ cup cooked diced potatoes

¼ teaspoon salt
⅛ teaspoon ground red pepper
2 teaspoons olive oil
1 tablespoon minced onion
 (1 teaspoon dried)
1 garlic clove, minced

1. Whisk the eggs and egg whites together in a medium bowl. Add the collards, potatoes, salt, and pepper and set aside.

2. Coat a medium nonstick skillet with vegetable oil spray; add the oil and heat over medium-high heat. Stir in the onion and garlic; cook 30 seconds. Whisk the egg mixture again and pour evenly into the skillet. Reduce the heat to medium and cook, without stirring, until the bottom is set and lightly browned, 3 to 4 minutes.*

3. Carefully slide the tortilla onto a large plate. Invert the skillet on top of the plate and, with oven mitts on both hands, turn the plate and skillet over together, flipping the tortilla back into the skillet. Cook until the eggs are set and the underside is lightly browned. Serve warm or at room temperature.

SERVES 2

*If you aren't confident about sliding and inverting the tortilla, there is another cooking method. Preheat the broiler. Add the oil to a flameproof skillet. Follow steps 1 and 2. When the bottom of the eggs is set and the top is still wet, place the skillet under the broiler and cook just until the tortilla top is set, about 2 minutes.

**Variation:** Spinach and Mushroom Tortilla: Substitute spinach for collard greens and mushrooms for potatoes. Coat a medium skillet with vegetable oil spray. Add the oil and heat over medium-high heat. Cook the mushrooms, stirring occasionally, until browned, about 3 minutes. Add the onion and garlic and cook 1 minute longer, stirring constantly. Pour the spinach-egg mixture into the vegetables in the skillet and follow the cooking instructions.

**Kilocalories 311 Kc • Protein 22 Gm • Fat 15 Gm • Percent of calories from fat 43% • Cholesterol 424 mg • Dietary Fiber 1 Gm • Sodium 550 mg • Calcium 372 mg**

# Spinach Scramble

*Perfect for a light dinner and it takes less than 10 minutes to cook. Serve with toasted challah or sourdough bread and sliced ripe tomatoes sprinkled with a few drops of balsamic vinegar.*

2 large eggs
3 egg whites
¼ teaspoon salt
¼ teaspoon freshly ground
  pepper

1 cup (packed) chopped fresh
  spinach
¼ cup crumbled feta cheese
1 tablespoon chopped fresh dill
1 teaspoon vegetable oil

1. Whisk the eggs, whites, salt, and pepper together in a medium bowl. Stir in the spinach, cheese, and dill.

2. Coat a medium skillet with vegetable oil spray. Add the oil and heat over medium-low heat. Add the spinach mixture and stir frequently until the eggs are cooked, 2 to 3 minutes. Serve immediately.

SERVES 2

**Kilocalories 210 Kc • Protein 17 Gm • Fat 14 Gm • Percent of calories from fat 61% • Cholesterol 240 mg • Dietary Fiber 1 Gm • Sodium 813 mg • Calcium 213 mg**

# Napa Cabbage and Bamboo Shoots in Black Bean Sauce (Microwave)

*This recipe is an easy and fast lunch dish. Served over cooked rice or couscous, it makes a delicious light dinner.*

2 tablespoons fermented black bean sauce

2 cups shredded napa or Chinese cabbage

1 can (8 ounces) bamboo shoots, drained

4 ounces firm tofu, drained and cut into bite-size cubes

1. Combine the black bean sauce with 1 tablespoon water in a small bowl.

2. Place the cabbage in a microwave-safe bowl; pour the black bean mixture over the cabbage. Cover with a lid or vented plastic wrap. Microwave on High for 3 minutes. Stir in the bamboo shoots and tofu and microwave on High for 2 minutes longer. Serve immediately.

SERVES 2

Kilocalories 90 Kc • Protein 9 Gm • Fat 3 Gm • Percent of calories from fat 29% • Cholesterol 0 mg • Dietary Fiber 4 Gm • Sodium 191 mg • Calcium 88 mg

# Lemon Pepper Shrimp (Microwave)

8 ounces jumbo frozen cooked
   shrimp
4 cups finely shredded iceberg
   lettuce or cabbage
2 tablespoons dry white wine or
   chicken broth

1 tablespoon peanut oil
2 large garlic cloves, minced
1 teaspoon mustard seed
½ teaspoon lemon pepper

1. Place the shrimp in a colander and run under cold water. Let them stand 1 hour.

2. Place the lettuce or cabbage in a microwave-safe shallow dish or pie plate. Add the wine and top with the shrimp. Cover with vented plastic wrap and microwave on High for 3 minutes.

3. Combine the oil, garlic, mustard seed, and pepper in a small skillet. Cook over low heat for 5 minutes. Drizzle the garlic mixture over the shrimp mixture and serve.

SERVES 2

Kilocalories 249 Kc • Protein 25 Gm • Fat 14 Gm • Percent of calories from fat 51% • Cholesterol 0 mg • Dietary Fiber 2 Gm • Sodium 802 mg • Calcium 129 mg

# Mom's Italian Spinach Sandwiches

2 tablespoons olive oil
4 large garlic cloves, thinly sliced
2 pounds spinach, trimmed,
    washed (do not dry), and
    coarsely chopped

1 teaspoon salt
2 loaves unsliced Italian bread
½ teaspoon red pepper flakes,
    optional

1. Heat 1 tablespoon of the oil in a large, deep pot or Dutch oven over medium heat. Add the garlic and cook about 30 seconds or until lightly browned.

2. Stir in the spinach and salt with ½ cup water. Cover and cook, stirring occasionally, for 15 minutes, until wilted.

3. Cut the bread crosswise into four 5-inch pieces (save any remaining bread for another use). Slice each piece horizontally, but not quite through the bread, starting on one long side, and open. Spoon the spinach mixture onto each bottom slice, drizzle with the remaining 1 tablespoon oil and sprinkle with the red pepper, if desired. Press the bread together and serve immediately.

SERVES 4

Kilocalories 480 Kc • Protein 18 Gm • Fat 11 Gm • Percent of calories from fat 20%
• Cholesterol 1 mg • Dietary Fiber 9 Gm • Sodium 1108 mg • Calcium 300 mg

# Grilled Pepper, Watercress, and Pepato Cheese Sandwich

*I used hydroponic (grown in water) spicy watercress, which I found in a specialty food store. It is a larger-leafed, very tender watercress with a peppery taste. To complement this green, I also used pepato cheese, which is a sheep's milk cheese studded with black peppercorns. Until recently this imported Sicilian cheese could only be found at gourmet food shops, but it is now made in Wisconsin and is available at most supermarkets.*

2 small red or yellow bell peppers
Salt
2 (5-inch) kaiser rolls, split
1 cup (lightly packed) spicy
    watercress leaves

2 teaspoons extra-virgin olive oil
½ cup (about 1½ ounces) slivered
    pepato cheese (black
    peppercorn cheese)

1. Preheat the broiler.

2. Cut the peppers in half and remove their seeds. Place them cut side down on a rack in a pan; coat with vegetable oil spray. Broil 1 inch from the heat for 5 minutes, until charred. Place the pan on a hot pad and cover the peppers with foil for 5 minutes.

3. Place 2 pepper halves on the bottom of each roll, cutting to fit, if necessary, and sprinkle with salt to taste. Top with the watercress and drizzle with the oil. Arrange the cheese on the watercress and cover with the top bread slices.

SERVES 2

Kilocalories 349 Kc • Protein 15 Gm • Fat 14 Gm • Percent of calories from fat 36% • Cholesterol 20 mg • Dietary Fiber 0 Gm • Sodium 501 mg • Calcium 295 mg

# Hot Dogs with Fresh Mustard Green Relish

*The relish may be made ahead and refrigerated. If you do lots of summer entertaining, double the recipe.*

4 cups coarsely chopped fresh mustard greens
1 small red bell pepper, seeded and coarsely chopped
½ medium Vidalia onion, coarsely chopped
1 cup apple cider vinegar
¼ cup sugar

¼ teaspoon ground cloves
¼ teaspoon ground cinnamon
⅛ teaspoon dry mustard
⅛ teaspoon salt
½ cup crushed canned pineapple with juice
6 turkey or meatless hot dogs
6 hot dog rolls

1. Place the greens, peppers, and onions in the bowl of a food processor. Process until minced.

2. Combine the vinegar and sugar in a medium saucepan (not aluminum). Bring to a boil, stirring to dissolve the sugar. Reduce the heat and stir in the cloves, cinnamon, mustard, and salt.

3. Simmer the mixture, uncovered, stirring frequently until the liquid is reduced slightly, about 20 minutes. Increase the heat to high and stir in the pineapple and juice. Cook 10 minutes longer, stirring frequently until thickened and syrupy. Cool at least 1 hour.

4. Preheat the grill according to manufacturer's instructions.

5. Cook the hot dogs to your liking. Open the rolls and toast for a minute or two on the grill. Place each hot dog in a roll, top with the relish, and serve immediately.

SERVES 6 (WITH ¼ CUP RELISH)

Kilocalories 233 Kc • Protein 12 Gm • Fat 2 Gm • Percent of calories from fat 9% • Cholesterol 15 mg • Dietary Fiber 1 Gm • Sodium 759 mg • Calcium 101 mg

# Eggplant and Arugula on Garlic Bread

1 loaf seeded Italian bread
1 garlic clove, cut lengthwise
   in half
1 medium eggplant (about 1
   pound), trimmed and cut
   crosswise into ½-inch slices
2 medium tomatoes, cut into
   ¼-inch slices

2 tablespoons balsamic vinegar
½ teaspoon kosher or
   coarse salt
¼ cup grated Romano cheese
3 cups chopped arugula
2 teaspoons extra-virgin
   olive oil

1. Preheat the broiler.

2. Slice the bread in half lengthwise. Coat the cut sides with vegetable oil spray. Place on a baking sheet and broil 3 inches from the heat until lightly browned, about 30 seconds. Rub each side with the garlic; discard the garlic.

3. Arrange the eggplant in a single layer on a baking sheet coated with vegetable oil spray. Coat the eggplant slices with additional spray. Broil 3 inches from the heat for 5 minutes; turn each slice and broil 5 minutes longer until lightly browned.

4. Place the eggplant and tomato slices on the bottom half of the bread. Sprinkle the vinegar, salt, and cheese on top of the vegetables, top with the arugula, and drizzle with the oil. Cover with the top slice and cut into 4 sandwiches.

SERVES 4

Kilocalories 290 Kc • Protein 12 Gm • Fat 6 Gm • Percent of calories from fat 18% • Cholesterol 6 mg • Dietary Fiber 4 Gm • Sodium 853 mg • Calcium 99 mg

# Caramelized Onions and Arugula on Sourdough

4 cups thinly sliced onion
3 teaspoons olive oil
2 teaspoons sugar
1 loaf (about 12 ounces)
   sourdough bread (Italian or
   French bread may be
   substituted)

Kosher or coarse salt
Freshly ground pepper
1 cup (packed) chopped arugula

1. Combine the onion, 2 teaspoons of the oil, and the sugar in a large nonstick skillet. Cover and cook over low heat for 15 minutes. Uncover, turn the heat to medium-high and cook, stirring frequently, 5 to 10 minutes longer, until browned.

2. Slice the loaf horizontally, not cutting all the way through starting on one long side. Open the bread and press down to flatten. Spread the onions on the bottom half of the bread and sprinkle with salt and pepper. Sprinkle a layer of arugula over the onions and drizzle with the remaining 1 teaspoon of oil. Close the loaf and press down; slice into 4 sandwiches and serve.

SERVES 4

**Variation:** Eliminate the cooked onion. Place ½ cup very thinly sliced raw red onion over 2 cups arugula on the bread; cover with thin slices of white Cheddar cheese. Wrap in foil and heat in a 350° oven for 15 minutes. Serve immediately.

Kilocalories 333 Kc • Protein 9 Gm • Fat 6 Gm • Percent of calories from fat 17%
• Cholesterol 0 mg • Dietary Fiber 5 Gm • Sodium 523 mg • Calcium 104 mg

# Broccoli Raab and Turkey Sausage on Semolina

4 Italian-style turkey or meatless sausages (about 2 ounces each)
12 ounces broccoli raab, trimmed and chopped (about 8 cups)
1 loaf seeded semolina Italian bread, split horizontally and cut into 4 equal pieces

4 teaspoons extra-virgin olive oil
½ teaspoon salt
Red pepper flakes, optional

1. Cook the sausage over low heat in a medium nonstick skillet coated with vegetable oil spray for 15 minutes; turn occasionally.

2. Place the broccoli raab in a collapsible steamer basket set over simmering water in a wide saucepan. Cover and steam 5 minutes.

3. Cut the sausages lengthwise in half. Place each opened sausage on a bottom half of the bread; top with broccoli raab and drizzle each with 1 teaspoon oil. Season with salt and red pepper, if desired. Cover each with the top slice and serve immediately.

SERVES 4

**Variation:** Substitute escarole for the broccoli raab. When steaming the escarole, arrange 1 cup diced red or yellow peppers on top. Steam both at once for about 8 minutes or until the escarole is tender.

Kilocalories 409 Kc • Protein 20 Gm • Fat 14 Gm • Percent of calories from fat 31% • Cholesterol 31 mg • Dietary Fiber 7 Gm • Sodium 1324 mg • Calcium 281 mg

# Skillet Turkey and Greens

*I've used canned mixed greens in this recipe, which makes this a very fast, yet nutritious meal to prepare. You might want to serve this with lightly buttered noodles or brown rice.*

2 teaspoons vegetable oil
¼ cup chopped onion
1 (8-ounce) boneless turkey
   tenderloin, cut into 1-inch cubes
1 can (14½ ounces) stewed
   tomatoes

1 cup cooked corn kernels
1 can (14 ounces) chopped mixed
   greens, drained
2 tablespoons chopped fresh flat-
   leaf parsley

1. Heat the oil in a large nonstick skillet over medium-high heat. Add the onion and cook 1 minute.

2. Add the turkey to the skillet and cook 1 minute, stirring, until browned. Reduce the heat; stir in the tomatoes, corn, greens, and parsley. Simmer, covered, for 15 minutes. Serve immediately.

SERVES 2

Kilocalories 358 Kc • Protein 43 Gm • Fat 7 Gm • Percent of calories from fat 16%
• Cholesterol 94 mg • Dietary Fiber 8 Gm • Sodium 748 mg • Calcium 234 mg

# Vegetable Trio on a French Baguette

*Carrots, as well as leafy greens, are a rich source of beta-carotene. Cook up a bunch to have on hand and add to leafy salads and sandwiches.*

2 cups steamed diced carrots
1 cup (packed) chopped chicory
1 peeled, roasted red pepper, chopped
1 tablespoon drained capers
1 tablespoon red wine vinegar

2 teaspoons extra-virgin olive oil
½ teaspoon dried oregano
1 French baguette (about 22 inches long), cut into 4 equal pieces

1. Combine all of the ingredients except the bread in a medium bowl.

2. Slice the bread horizontally. Spoon equal amounts (about 1 cup) of the vegetable mixture on the bottom of each bread slice; cover with the top slice and serve.

SERVES 4

Kilocalories 300 Kc  •  Protein 9 Gm  •  Fat 5 Gm  •  Percent of calories from fat 15%  •  Cholesterol 0 mg  •  Dietary Fiber 5 Gm  •  Sodium 636 mg  •  Calcium 132 mg

# Tuna-Vegetable Baguette Sandwich

*This sandwich may be made the night before for a delicious desk-top lunch. Just mound about ¾ cup of the filling onto the bottom slice of bread, top with the remaining slice, and press down. Wrap the sandwich in foil and refrigerate.*

1 can (6 ounces) tuna in water, drained
1½ cups finely chopped romaine lettuce
2 tablespoons grated onion
2 tablespoons sliced pimiento olives
2 tablespoons shredded carrot
1 tablespoon red wine vinegar
2 teaspoons extra-virgin olive oil
½ teaspoon dried tarragon
1 French baguette (about 22 inches long), cut into 4 equal pieces

1. Combine all of the ingredients except the baguette in a medium bowl.

2. Slice the bread horizontally. Spoon equal amounts of the tuna mixture on the bottom of each bread slice, cover with the top slice, and serve.

SERVES 4

Kilocalories 272 Kc • Protein 19 Gm • Fat 4 Gm • Percent of calories from fat 15%
• Cholesterol 13 mg • Dietary Fiber 1 Gm • Sodium 685 mg • Calcium 25 mg

# Turkey Divan (Microwave)

*Broccoli has been eliminated in this classic dish and replaced with spinach. Fresh apple or cranberry sauce is a good accompaniment.*

2 tablespoons unsalted butter
3 tablespoons all-purpose flour
1 cup chicken broth
1 teaspoon chopped fresh
    tarragon leaves (¼ teaspoon
    dried)

⅛ teaspoon freshly ground
    pepper
1 package (10 ounces) frozen
    chopped spinach, thawed,
    drained, and squeezed
12 ounces sliced cooked turkey

1. Place the butter in a 4-cup glass measure. Microwave on High for 30 seconds, until melted. Stir in the flour and microwave on High for 30 seconds longer.

2. Gradually whisk in the broth, tarragon, and pepper. Microwave on High for 1 minute. Whisk vigorously and microwave on High for 1 to 2 minutes longer, until thickened, stirring once.

3. Spoon the spinach into a 9-inch microwave-safe pie plate. Arrange the turkey slices on top and drizzle with the sauce. Cover with vented plastic wrap and microwave on Medium-High for 3 minutes, turning the dish once during the cooking. Let it stand 1 minute and serve.

SERVES 2

Kilocalories 416 Kc • Protein 58 Gm • Fat 12 Gm • Percent of calories from fat 27%
• Cholesterol 168 mg • Dietary Fiber 5 Gm • Sodium 258 mg • Calcium 250 mg

# Roasted Tofu with Green Caper Sauce

*Be sure to serve the tofu straight from the oven or it gets tough.*

¼ cup (packed) arugula leaves
¼ cup (packed) fresh basil leaves
¼ cup vegetable broth or water
1½ tablespoons olive oil
1 tablespoon capers, drained

⅛ teaspoon freshly ground
  pepper
1 pound firm tofu, drained and
  dried with paper towels

1. Preheat the oven to 500°.

2. Puree the arugula, basil, broth or water, oil, capers, and pepper in a small food processor. Pour into a small saucepan and keep warm over very low heat.

3. With a large knife, cut the tofu horizontally in 4 slices. Place on a baking sheet coated with vegetable oil spray. Coat the tops of the tofu with additional spray. Roast about 20 minutes until slightly browned and sizzling.

4. With a spatula, carefully place one tofu slice on each of 4 serving plates. Drizzle the sauce over evenly. Serve immediately.

SERVES 4

Kilocalories 117 Kc • Protein 9 Gm • Fat 8 Gm • Percent of calories from fat 57%
• Cholesterol 0 mg • Dietary Fiber 0 Gm • Sodium 157 mg • Calcium 48 mg

# Spinach Fettuccine and Vegetables

6 ounces spinach fettuccine
2 tablespoons olive oil
2 cups halved, trimmed fresh
 mushrooms
1 cup cherry tomatoes, halved
1 cup chopped fresh spinach
3 tablespoons dry vermouth or
 vegetable broth

1½ cups part-skim ricotta cheese
½ cup grated Romano cheese
 (about 2 ounces)
¼ cup skim milk
¼ teaspoon freshly ground
 pepper
2 tablespoons chopped fresh flat-
 leaf parsley

1. Cook the pasta according to the package directions. Drain well.

2. Meanwhile, heat the oil in a medium nonstick skillet over medium-high heat. Add the mushrooms and tomatoes and cook for 1 to 2 minutes, stirring occasionally, until the mushrooms are lightly browned. Reduce the heat and stir in the spinach and vermouth. Cook 1 minute.

3. Combine the ricotta, Romano cheese, milk, and pepper in a serving bowl. Stir in the vegetable mixture and the cooked pasta. Sprinkle with the parsley and serve immediately.

SERVES 2

Kilocalories 890 Kc • Protein 47 Gm • Fat 40 Gm • Percent of calories from fat 40%
• Cholesterol 168 mg • Dietary Fiber 9 Gm • Sodium 685 mg • Calcium 934 mg

# Vegetable Risotto

*This risotto is intended as a main course for a light meal.*

2 cups chicken broth
1 tablespoon olive oil
½ cup chopped red onion
2 cups chopped zucchini
2 cups chopped savoy
   cabbage

1 cup arborio rice
⅛ teaspoon ground saffron
1 tablespoon (packed)
   shredded fresh basil
   leaves
Salt and freshly ground pepper

1. In a medium saucepan, simmer the broth and 1 cup water over low heat.

2. Heat the oil in a Dutch oven over medium heat. Add the onion and cook about 3 minutes, stirring frequently, until tender.

3. Add the zucchini and cabbage to the onion. Cover and cook 5 minutes, stirring occasionally, until softened.

4. Stir the rice and saffron into the vegetable mixture. Using a ladle or measuring cup, add about ½ cup of the hot broth to the rice mixture. Cook, stirring constantly, until the liquid is fully absorbed, about 5 minutes. Repeat, adding ½ cup liquid at a time, until the rice is just tender and creamy, about 20 minutes. Stir in the basil and season with salt and pepper to taste. Serve immediately.

SERVES 3

Kilocalories 381 Kc • Protein 9 Gm • Fat 6 Gm • Percent of calories from fat 16%
• Cholesterol 3 mg • Dietary Fiber 4 Gm • Sodium 78 mg • Calcium 36 mg

# Bok Choy, Chicken, and Walnuts

3 tablespoons dry sherry or chicken broth

2 tablespoons hoisin sauce

1 skinless, boneless chicken breast (about 8 ounces), cut into 1-inch cubes

1 tablespoon peanut oil

1 small bunch bok choy (about 1 pound), trimmed and chopped

½ teaspoon salt

1 teaspoon cornstarch

2 tablespoons coarsely chopped walnuts

1. Whisk the sherry and hoisin sauce together in a shallow bowl; add the chicken and let it stand 30 minutes, stirring occasionally, at room temperature.

2. Heat the oil over high heat in a wok or skillet. Remove the chicken from the marinade (reserve the marinade) with a large slotted spoon and add to the wok. Cook for 3 to 4 minutes until browned and cooked through. Remove with a slotted spoon to a dish.

3. Add the bok choy and salt to the wok; cook 5 minutes, stirring frequently, until browned and wilted. Add to the chicken in the dish.

4. While the bok choy is cooking, whisk the cornstarch and ¼ cup water into the reserved marinade until smooth. Stir the marinade into the wok and cook, stirring constantly, 1 minute. Stir in the chicken and bok choy and cook 1 minute longer or until heated through. Sprinkle with the walnuts and serve immediately.

SERVES 2

Kilocalories 400 Kc • Protein 41 Gm • Fat 18 Gm • Percent of calories from fat 41% • Cholesterol 96 mg • Dietary Fiber 2 Gm • Sodium 709 mg • Calcium 216 mg

# Salad in a Pocket

*I love peanut butter! In this recipe, it's used as a base for the dressing. These sandwiches are really stuffed, so they're a little messy to eat, but worth it. Wrap the bottom half of the sandwich in foil to eliminate dripping.*

*Dressing:*

½ cup smooth peanut butter
¼ cup plain nonfat yogurt
1½ tablespoons dark sesame oil

4 (6-inch) whole wheat pita
   breads

*Filling:*

2 cups shredded iceberg lettuce
1 cup nonfat cottage cheese
1 cup shredded low-fat Cheddar
   cheese (about 4 ounces)
½ cup shredded carrot
½ cup diced tomato

1. To prepare the dressing, whisk the peanut butter, yogurt, and oil together in a 1-cup measure.

2. Slit the top of each pita with a knife. Push ½ cup lettuce to the bottom of each pita. Spoon ¼ cup cottage cheese over the lettuce, then equal amounts of the Cheddar, carrot, and tomato. Drizzle the dressing into each pita and serve.

SERVES 4

**Variation:** Dressing: ½ cup plain nonfat yogurt, 4 teaspoons dark sesame oil, 2 teaspoons fresh chopped cilantro. Filling: 2 cups tat soi instead of lettuce, shredded Monterey Jack cheese instead of Cheddar, and diced green bell pepper instead of carrot.

Kilocalories 502 Kc • Protein 34 Gm • Fat 25 Gm • Percent of calories from fat 42% • Cholesterol 15 mg • Dietary Fiber 8 Gm • Sodium 753 mg • Calcium 442 mg

# Pita Pockets with Cobb Salad

2 tablespoons vegetable oil
1 tablespoon red wine vinegar
¼ teaspoon salt
¼ teaspoon freshly ground
  pepper
2 cups diced cooked chicken or
  cubed, drained firm tofu
1 small avocado, peeled, pitted,
  and finely chopped

½ cup diced cooked beets (if
  using canned, drain well)
½ cup diced ripe tomato
½ cup crumbled blue cheese
  (about 2 ounces)
4 (7-inch) pitas
2 cups shredded romaine lettuce
1 hard-cooked large egg, finely
  chopped

1. Combine the oil, vinegar, salt, and pepper with 1 tablespoon water in a medium bowl. Add the chicken, avocado, beets, tomato, and cheese and toss lightly.

2. Cut the pita loaves in half crosswise. Stuff each half with equal amounts of the lettuce and the chicken mixture. Sprinkle with the egg and serve.

SERVES 4

Kilocalories 519 Kc • Protein 34 Gm • Fat 25 Gm • Percent of calories from fat 42%
• Cholesterol 123 mg • Dietary Fiber 6 Gm • Sodium 842 mg • Calcium 124 mg

# Focaccia Sandwich with Arugula and Fontina Cheese

*Focaccia is an ancient flatbread dating back to Neolithic times. Carbonized remnants have been found in the ruins of many countries bordering the Mediterranean. Often I am asked, what makes focaccia different from pizza? Not much, except for the topping.*

2 slices (4 inches wide) focaccia bread, split
2 ounces thinly sliced fontina cheese, rind removed
2 teaspoons chopped fresh sage (do not use dried)

1 cup arugula leaves (not packed)
4 thin slices tomato
2 teaspoons balsamic or sherry vinegar
¼ teaspoon freshly ground pepper

1. Preheat the oven to 300°.
2. Place the cheese on the bottom slices of bread; sprinkle with the sage. Top with the arugula and tomato. Sprinkle each half with vinegar and pepper. Cover with the top slice. Wrap each sandwich in foil and bake 15 minutes.

SERVES 2

**Variation:** Spread each bottom slice with 2 teaspoons prepared pesto; top with thin slices of smoked mozzarella (about 2 ounces for each) and red onion. Top each sandwich with ½ cup baby spinach. Drizzle each with 1 teaspoon red wine vinegar. Sprinkle with salt and pepper, if desired.

Kilocalories 438 Kc • Protein 22 Gm • Fat 16 Gm • Percent of calories from fat 32% • Cholesterol 42 mg • Dietary Fiber 1 Gm • Sodium 856 mg • Calcium 374 mg

# Mess o' Greens Sandwich

*This is a spinach-packed, hearty sandwich. For a light dinner, serve it with a baked potato or, if you're living dangerously, French fries.*

½ cup part-skim ricotta cheese
1 teaspoon lemon pepper
2 seeded kaiser rolls, split

1 package (10 ounces) frozen leaf spinach, cooked, drained, squeezed, and coarsely chopped

Combine the ricotta and lemon pepper in a small bowl. Spread the top slice of each roll with the cheese mixture. Place 1 cup spinach on the bottom half of each roll, cover with the top slices and serve.

SERVES 2

Kilocalories 257 Kc • Protein 15 Gm • Fat 4 Gm • Percent of calories from fat 15% • Cholesterol 8 mg • Dietary Fiber 5 Gm • Sodium 478 mg • Calcium 339 mg

# Spinach and Feta Burritos

*When you have a cup of leftover cooked greens, think of these burritos.*

1 cup coarsely chopped cooked spinach

¼ cup crumbled feta cheese with black pepper
2 (7-inch) flour tortillas

1. Preheat the oven to 300°.
2. Spoon ½ cup spinach down the center of each tortilla. Top each with 2 tablespoons of feta cheese. Fold left and right sides of the tortilla toward the center, overlapping the edges. Wrap in foil and bake 10 minutes.

SERVES 2

Kilocalories 224 Kc • Protein 11 Gm • Fat 9 Gm • Percent of calories from fat 37% • Cholesterol 28 mg • Dietary Fiber 4 Gm • Sodium 603 mg • Calcium 339 mg

# Stuffed French Toast

*A side of baked chips and a pickle is perfect for this grilled cheese alternative.*

1 package (10 ounces) frozen
  turnip greens
¼ cup chopped onion
1 cup vegetable broth or water
6 slices multi-grain bread
6 very thin slices tomato

3 teaspoons vegetable oil
¾ cup thawed egg substitute or
  3 large eggs
¼ teaspoon salt
⅛ teaspoon cayenne pepper
⅛ teaspoon dry mustard

1. Combine the turnip greens and onion with the broth in a medium saucepan. Bring to a boil, separating the frozen block with a fork. Reduce the heat, cover, and cook for 15 minutes. Drain, cool, and squeeze out the excess liquid. Spread a heaping ¼ cup greens mixture on each of 3 slices of bread; top with the tomato slices and cover each with another slice of bread.

2. Coat a large nonstick skillet with vegetable oil spray. Add 2 teaspoons of the oil and heat over medium heat.

3. Whisk the egg substitute, salt, cayenne, and dry mustard together in a shallow dish. Dip the sandwich in the egg mixture, carefully turning over to coat the other side. Place in the prepared skillet. Cook the sandwich about 2 minutes on each side, until lightly browned. Place on a large serving plate and cover with foil to keep warm.

4. Add the remaining teaspoon of oil to the skillet. Repeat the process with the remaining 2 sandwiches. Cut the sandwiches in half on the diagonal and serve immediately.

SERVES 3

Kilocalories 308 Kc • Protein 15 Gm • Fat 14 Gm • Percent of calories from fat 39%
• Cholesterol 1 mg • Dietary Fiber 5 Gm • Sodium 762 mg • Calcium 227 mg

# Pita Calzone

*The word* calzoni *means "pant legs" in Italian. These half-moon–shaped turnovers, usually filled with cheese and meats, were originally shaped more like tubes. While they baked, the dough puffed up much like the billowing trousers of eighteenth-century Neapolitan men.*

1 cup part-skim ricotta cheese
½ cup finely chopped arugula
½ cup chopped drained pimiento
⅓ cup shredded part-skim
   mozzarella

2 tablespoons grated Romano
   cheese
4 (1-ounce) whole wheat pita
   breads

1. To make the filling, combine all of the ingredients, except the bread, in a medium bowl. Cover and refrigerate 3 hours or overnight.

2. Preheat the oven to 350°.

3. Slit one end of each pita to make an opening. Spoon a heaping ⅓ cup filling into each pita. Wrap each in foil and bake for 20 to 25 minutes, until heated through.

SERVES 4

Kilocalories 215 Kc • Protein 14 Gm • Fat 9 Gm • Percent of calories from fat 36%
• Cholesterol 31 mg • Dietary Fiber 2 Gm • Sodium 382 mg • Calcium 248 mg

# Grilled Chicken and Watercress on Wheat

1 cup egg substitute
2 teaspoons snipped fresh dill (½ teaspoon dried)
1 can (4 ounces) water-packed chunk white chicken, drained

⅓ cup finely chopped watercress
3 tablespoons light mayonnaise
2 teaspoons minced onion
8 slices whole wheat bread
2 teaspoons vegetable oil

1. Combine the egg substitute and dill in a shallow dish and set aside.

2. Combine the chicken, watercress, mayonnaise, and onion in a small bowl. Spread one fourth of the mixture on 4 slices of bread; cover each with a top slice.

3. Coat a large nonstick skillet with vegetable oil spray. Add the oil and heat over medium heat.

4. Dip each sandwich into the egg mixture, turning to coat both sides. Cook 3 to 5 minutes on each side until golden. Serve immediately.

SERVES 4

Kilocalories 274 Kc • Protein 18 Gm • Fat 12 Gm • Percent of calories from fat 38%
• Cholesterol 18 mg • Dietary Fiber 4 Gm • Sodium 553 mg • Calcium 73 mg

# Sweet and Savory Cream Cheese on Raisin Toast

*For a chunky texture, use a crisp Bosc pear, but if you prefer a creamier spread, use a ripe Bartlett or Comice pear.*

4 ounces light cream cheese
½ cup finely chopped arugula

1 ripe pear, peeled, cored, and finely chopped
8 slices cinnamon raisin bread

1. Combine the cheese, arugula, and pear in a small bowl. Cover and refrigerate until ready to use.

2. Toast the bread. Spread a heaping ¼ cup of the cream cheese mixture on each of 4 slices of toast. Cover with the remaining slices and serve.

SERVES 4

**Variation:** Substitute 1 Red or Golden Delicious apple for the pear and add 2 teaspoons apple butter to the spread.

Kilocalories 230 Kc • Protein 7 Gm • Fat 7 Gm • Percent of calories from fat 27% • Cholesterol 13 mg • Dietary Fiber 3 Gm • Sodium 336 mg • Calcium 78 mg

# Cream Cheese and Spinach Rollup Sandwiches (Toaster Oven)

8 slices soft white or whole wheat bread
8 tablespoons light cream cheese, softened
2 teaspoons lemon pepper
1 cup minced fresh spinach
Apple or pear slices, optional

1. Preheat the toaster oven to 350°.

2. Trim the crusts from the bread. With a rolling pin, roll each slice as thinly as possible.

3. Spread each slice of bread with 1 tablespoon cream cheese. Sprinkle each with ¼ teaspoon lemon pepper and 2 tablespoons spinach. Roll each slice up and press down to seal. Place in the toaster oven and bake 5 minutes. Serve with apples or pears, if desired.

SERVES 4

Kilocalories 210 Kc • Protein 8 Gm • Fat 7 Gm • Percent of calories from fat 31% • Cholesterol 15 mg • Dietary Fiber 2 Gm • Sodium 420 mg • Calcium 122 mg

# Chicken Cutlets, Sun-Dried Tomatoes, and Arugula Mayonnaise

1 cup sun-dried tomatoes
¼ cup minced arugula
¼ cup light mayonnaise
¼ cup plain dried bread crumbs
3 tablespoons skim milk

4 very thin chicken cutlets (about 6 ounces)
1 loaf whole wheat Italian bread, cut into 4 pieces

1. Preheat the oven to 400°.

2. Combine the tomatoes with 1 cup boiling water in a medium bowl. Let them stand 10 minutes, drain, and coarsely chop.

3. Combine the arugula and mayonnaise in a small bowl. Refrigerate, covered, until ready to use.

4. Place the bread crumbs on wax paper and pour the milk into a small dish. Dip the cutlets in the milk, then coat them with the crumbs. Place on a baking sheet coated with vegetable oil spray. Bake 6 minutes, turn, and bake 6 minutes longer or until done.

5. Cut the bread slices horizontally. Place 1 chicken cutlet on the bottom half of each slice; top each with ¼ of the tomatoes. Spread the mayonnaise mixture on the top slices, cover, and press the sandwiches together. Serve immediately.

SERVES 4

Kilocalories 587 Kc • Protein 64 Gm • Fat 13 Gm • Percent of calories from fat 21% • Cholesterol 146 mg • Dietary Fiber 3 Gm • Sodium 1046 mg • Calcium 72 mg

# Escarole Frittata on Focaccia

4 large eggs
4 egg whites
1 teaspoon dried oregano
¾ teaspoon salt
½ teaspoon freshly ground
  pepper

2 cups (packed) finely shredded
  escarole (wet)
1 cup diced red bell pepper
1 tablespoon grated Romano
  cheese
4 slices (4 inches wide) focaccia
  bread

1. Whisk the eggs, whites, oregano, salt, and ground pepper together in a medium bowl and set aside.

2. Preheat the broiler. (If your nonstick skillet is not ovenproof, wrap the handle in a triple thickness of foil before broiling.)

3. Combine the escarole and bell peppers with ¼ cup water in a large nonstick skillet coated with vegetable oil spray. Cover and cook over medium heat for 5 minutes. Uncover, stir, and add the egg mixture.

4. Reduce the heat and cook the eggs for 3 to 4 minutes, or until the eggs are set around the edge and light brown on the bottom. Sprinkle with the cheese and broil 5 inches from the heat about 2 minutes or until golden brown.

5. Slice the focaccia horizontally. Cut the frittata in quarters. Fold each to fit on the bottom half of the focaccia. Cover with the top slices and serve.

SERVES 4

Kilocalories 264 Kc • Protein 19 Gm • Fat 11 Gm • Percent of calories from fat 37%
• Cholesterol 221 mg • Dietary Fiber 3 Gm • Sodium 1081 mg • Calcium 193 mg

# Pumpernickel with Spinach Spread and Tomatoes

*This nonfat spread is a good alternative to mayonnaise. You can add any seasonings that you like.*

½ cup coarsely chopped fresh
   spinach
¾ cup nonfat cottage cheese
1 teaspoon spicy brown mustard
¼ teaspoon salt

⅛ teaspoon freshly ground
   pepper
8 slices pumpernickel bread
8 (¼-inch) tomato slices (about
   2 medium tomatoes)

1. Mince the spinach in a small food processor. Add the cottage cheese, mustard, salt, and pepper; process until smooth.

2. Spread the cheese mixture on each slice of bread. Top 4 of the bread slices with 2 tomatoes slices each, and cover with the remaining bread, cheese side down. Serve immediately.

SERVES 4

Kilocalories 206 Kc • Protein 12 Gm • Fat 2 Gm • Percent of calories from fat 10% • Cholesterol 4 mg • Dietary Fiber 5 Gm • Sodium 741 mg • Calcium 77 mg

# Zucchini Rolls Stuffed with Ricotta and Mizuna

*A great way to use up that bumper summer crop of zucchini.*

3 medium zucchini
1½ cups (packed) mizuna
10 large fresh basil
    leaves
1 cup plus 2 tablespoons part-
    skim ricotta cheese

2 tablespoons light cream
    cheese
⅛ teaspoon salt
⅛ teaspoon freshly ground
    pepper
1 cup marinara sauce, preferably
    homemade

1. Preheat the oven to 500°.

2. Cut the zucchini lengthwise into twelve ¼-inch-thick slices (save any extra zucchini for salads). Coat a baking sheet with vegetable oil spray. Place the zucchini on the sheet and coat lightly with additional spray. Roast for 10 minutes. Place the pan on a rack and cool.

3. Mince ½ cup of the mizuna and basil in a small food processor. Add the ricotta, cream cheese, salt, and pepper and process for 10 seconds until smooth. Let the mixture stand at room temperature for 30 minutes.

4. Heat the marinara sauce in a small saucepan over low heat.

5. Place a tablespoonful of the filling on the wider end of each zucchini slice and roll. Arrange ¼ cup of the remaining mizuna on each of 4 plates; stand 3 zucchini rolls upright on top. Drizzle with the sauce and serve.

SERVES 4

Kilocalories 165 Kc • Protein 11 Gm • Fat 9 Gm • Percent of calories from fat 48% • Cholesterol 26 mg • Dietary Fiber 3 Gm • Sodium 436 mg • Calcium 232 mg

# Marjatta's Spinach Crepes

*Marjatta, a friend from Finland, calls crepes "pancakes." She always has them on hand because they freeze very well. After the crepes are completely cooled, stack each one between layers of wax paper. Wrap in aluminum foil and freeze. Defrost at room temperature. Unfilled, these crepes are a great substitute for rice, potato, or pasta side dishes.*

1 cup all-purpose flour
1 cup 1% milk
2 large eggs
1 tablespoon unsalted butter, melted
½ teaspoon salt

½ package (10 ounces) frozen chopped spinach, thawed, drained, and squeezed
Grated Parmesan cheese, optional

1. Preheat the oven to the warm setting.

2. Whisk the flour, milk, eggs, butter, and salt together in a medium bowl. Whisk in the spinach until combined.

3. Coat a crepe pan or an 8-inch nonstick sauté pan with vegetable oil spray. Heat the pan over medium-high heat until a drop of water sprinkled in the pan sizzles. For each crepe, pour a scant ¼ cup batter into the center of the pan, spreading with a spoon until a thin film covers the bottom. Cook 1 to 2 minutes or until the underside is light brown and dry. Run a spatula around the edges and lift out. Turn and cook about 30 seconds longer.

4. Sprinkle each crepe with a little Parmesan cheese and roll. Cover with foil and place in the oven until ready to serve.

SERVES 6 (2 CREPES EACH)

**Variation:** Swiss Cheese Crepes: Preheat the broiler. Coat an 11 × 7 × 2-inch baking pan with vegetable oil spray. Roll up the crepes and place side by side, seam side down, in the pan. Sprinkle evenly with 1 cup (4 ounces) shredded Swiss cheese. Broil 2 inches from the heat until the cheese is melted, about 2 minutes.

**Kilocalories 149 Kc • Protein 7 Gm • Fat 4 Gm • Percent of calories from fat 26% • Cholesterol 78 mg • Dietary Fiber 2 Gm • Sodium 277 mg • Calcium 151 mg**

# Herbed Eggplant and Spinach Rollatine

1 medium eggplant (about 1 pound), trimmed and cut into eight ¼-inch lengthwise slices
2½ tablespoons olive oil
1 tablespoon balsamic vinegar
1 tablespoon chopped fresh thyme (½ teaspoon dried)
1 tablespoon chopped fresh oregano (½ teaspoon dried)
1 tablespoon chopped fresh mint

1 tablespoon chopped fresh basil (½ teaspoon dried)
¼ teaspoon salt

*Filling:*

½ cup cooked, drained, and chopped spinach
½ cup part-skim ricotta cheese
¼ teaspoon salt
⅛ teaspoon freshly grated nutmeg
Fresh herbs for garnish

1. Blanch the eggplant in a large pot of simmering water for 3 minutes. Drain on paper towels.

2. Combine 2 tablespoons of the oil, the vinegar, herbs, and ¼ teaspoon salt in a 13×9-inch baking dish. Add the eggplant, turning to coat; marinate in the refrigerator overnight, turning occasionally. Remove from the refrigerator and let the dish stand at room temperature 1 hour.

3. To prepare the filling, whisk the spinach, ricotta, salt, and the nutmeg together in a medium bowl until smooth. Spread about 3 tablespoons of the spinach mixture over each eggplant slice; roll up.

4. Place 2 eggplant rolls on each of 4 plates. Drizzle with the remaining ½ tablespoon olive oil. Garnish with herbs.

SERVES 4

Kilocalories 158 Kc • Protein 5 Gm • Fat 11 Gm • Percent of calories from fat 61% • Cholesterol 10 mg • Dietary Fiber 1 Gm • Sodium 353 mg • Calcium 131 mg

# California Quesadillas

*My daughter, Jenna, is the quesadilla "queen." Her fascination began as a hungry student in L.A. A New Yorker by birth, she gave up East Coast citizenship when she tasted her first quesadilla. This California version of the Mexican original became the staple of her student diet, followed by the ubiquitous peanut butter and jelly sandwich and pizza.*

4 (8-inch) flour tortillas
1 cup shredded Monterey Jack cheese (4 ounces)

1 cup chopped mesclun
½ teaspoon ground cumin

1. Lay 2 tortillas on a flat surface. Sprinkle each with ¼ cup cheese to within 1 inch of the edge. Top each with ½ cup mesclun and sprinkle with the cumin. Top each with the remaining cheese and tortillas.

2. Coat a griddle with vegetable oil spray and place over medium heat. When the griddle is hot, place the quesadilla in the center, pressing down with a spatula. Cook 1 minute, turn carefully, and cook 1 minute longer. Repeat with the remaining quesadilla. Cut each quesadilla in quarters.

SERVES 2

**Variation:** For a more substantial quesadilla, add ½ cup finely chopped cooked chicken and 3 tablespoons salsa per quesadilla. These are a little bulkier to lift onto the griddle, so press them together first.

Kilocalories 436 Kc • Protein 19 Gm • Fat 23 Gm • Percent of calories from fat 47% • Cholesterol 60 mg • Dietary Fiber 3 Gm • Sodium 719 mg • Calcium 504 mg

# Corn Tortilla Quesadillas

*"Real" Mexican quesadillas are actually made with unbaked corn tortilla dough, according to one of my favorite cookbook authors and authority on Mexican food, Elizabeth Lambert Ortiz. The following quesadillas are a good light lunch, but if you cut each into 3 triangles and serve with salsa, they become delicious appetizers.*

4 (6-inch) corn tortillas
1 cup chopped mizuna or fresh
  spinach

1 cup Queso quesadilla cheese
  (or Monterey Jack)
¼ cup chopped fresh cilantro

1. Hold the tortilla in your hand folded in half. Fill each with one fourth each of the greens, cheese, and cilantro. Press tightly so the fold remains and the filling doesn't fall out.

2. Coat a griddle with vegetable oil spray and place over medium heat. When the griddle is hot, arrange as many of the quesadillas as you can in a single layer. Cook 1 minute, turn carefully, and cook 1 minute longer. Repeat for any uncooked quesadillas. Serve immediately.

SERVES 2

**Variation:** Baked Quesadilla: Preheat the oven to 400°. Combine ½ cup steamed broccoli raab, ¼ cup *each* part-skim ricotta and shredded mozzarella, ¼ teaspoon salt, and ⅛ teaspoon *each* red pepper flakes and garlic powder. Spread each of 2 tortillas with half the mixture and top each with another tortilla, lightly pressing together. Place on a baking sheet and cover with foil. Bake 3 to 5 minutes until the cheese begins to melt. Remove the foil and carefully turn the tortillas with a large spatula. Bake until crisp on top, about 2 minutes. Turn over again and bake until lightly browned on the other side, 1 to 2 minutes.

Kilocalories 409 Kc • Protein 19 Gm • Fat 19 Gm • Percent of calories from fat 41% • Cholesterol 54 mg • Dietary Fiber 5 Gm • Sodium 519 mg • Calcium 588 mg

# Easy Stuffed Cabbage Rolls

8 large outside cabbage leaves
2 teaspoons vegetable oil
8 ounces ground lean chicken
1 cup cooked white rice
2 tablespoons finely chopped
onion
2 teaspoons reduced-sodium soy
sauce

2 teaspoons Worcestershire
sauce
1 teaspoon soy bacon bits,
optional
1 teaspoon sugar
¼ teaspoon celery seeds
¼ teaspoon dried oregano
1 cup canned tomato sauce

1. Preheat the oven to 350°.

2. Bring a large pot of salted water to a boil. Drop the cabbage leaves into the water and boil for 4 minutes, or until the leaves are limp and pliable. Drain. (A small portion of the thick center rib may have to be removed in order to roll the leaves; try folding one leaf first.)

3. Heat the oil in a medium nonstick skillet over medium heat. Add the chicken and cook until no longer pink, stirring frequently, 3 to 5 minutes. Combine the chicken with the rice, onion, soy, Worcestershire, bacon bits, sugar, celery seeds, and oregano in a medium bowl.

4. Divide the mixture evenly among the cabbage leaves. Starting at the stem end of each leaf, roll the leaf around the mixture, tucking in the sides, envelope style.

5. Spoon half of the tomato sauce into a Dutch oven; arrange the cabbage rolls, seam side down, on top. Cover with the remaining tomato sauce. Bake, covered, 1 hour, or until tender.

SERVES 4

Kilocalories 341 Kc • Protein 23 Gm • Fat 5 Gm • Percent of calories from fat 14% • Cholesterol 48 mg • Dietary Fiber 3 Gm • Sodium 561 mg • Calcium 86 mg

# Scallops in Romaine

⅓ cup sliced scallions
1 tablespoon low-sodium soy
  sauce
2 teaspoons vegetable oil
⅛ teaspoon ground red
  pepper
1 pound sea scallops
½ cup semidry white wine such as
  a Reisling or Gewürztraminer

4 large romaine lettuce leaves
½ cup bottled clam juice
1 tablespoon distilled white
  vinegar
1 bay leaf
½ cup plain low-fat yogurt
½ cup diced red bell pepper

1. Combine the scallions, soy, oil, and ground pepper in a medium bowl. Add the scallops, cover, and refrigerate for 30 minutes.

2. Bring the wine to a simmer over medium heat in a large nonreactive, nonstick skillet. Add the lettuce and cover. Reduce the heat and cook for 3 minutes until the lettuce wilts. Remove with a slotted spoon, reserving the wine.

3. Spoon equal amounts of the scallop mixture onto the center of each leaf. Fold all 4 sides of the lettuce to cover the mixture, forming a packet.

4. Add the clam juice, vinegar, and bay leaf to the wine in the skillet; bring to a boil. Carefully place each lettuce packet, seam side down, in the skillet. Reduce the heat, cover, and simmer for 5 minutes. Remove from the heat and let the pot stand, covered, for 5 minutes. Remove the packets with a slotted spoon and place them on serving plates. Discard the bay leaf.

5. Bring the liquid in the skillet to a boil over medium-high heat; cook about 5 minutes or until reduced to 2 tablespoons. Remove from the heat and gradually whisk in the yogurt until the mixture is smooth. Spoon 2 tablespoons of the sauce over each packet and garnish with the bell pepper. Serve immediately.

SERVES 4

Kilocalories 176 Kc • Protein 24 Gm • Fat 4 Gm • Percent of calories from fat 21%
• Cholesterol 50 mg • Dietary Fiber 1 Gm • Sodium 487 mg • Calcium 175 mg

# Radicchio Bundles

*This is a colorful and tasty first course. Ackawi is a semi-soft Arabic cheese that is sold in Middle Eastern markets and some supermarkets. If you can't find it, use goat cheese as a substitute.*

1 large red bell pepper, seeded
   and cut into eighths
2 cups julienned zucchini
   (1 medium)
¼ teaspoon kosher salt
8 large radicchio leaves

1 teaspoon minced fresh
   marjoram (½ teaspoon dried)
½ cup crumbled Ackawi cheese
2 teaspoons extra-virgin
   olive oil
4 sprigs fresh marjoram for
   garnish

1. Preheat the oven to 500°F. Coat a baking sheet with vegetable oil spray.

2. Place the peppers, skin side down, on the prepared pan. Place the zucchini in the pan in one layer. Spray the vegetables with vegetable oil spray and sprinkle with salt. Roast 20 minutes until the vegetables are charred. Cool and coarsely chop the peppers.

3. Divide the peppers and zucchini among the radicchio leaves. Sprinkle the mixture with the minced majoram and cheese. Fold the leaves to close and secure them with toothpicks. Place, seam side up, on baking sheets. Brush with the oil. Roast 10 minutes. Place the rolls on serving plates and remove the toothpicks. Garnish the plates with sprigs of marjoram.

SERVES 4

Kilocalories 76 Kc • Protein 4 Gm • Fat 5 Gm • Percent of calories from fat 61% • Cholesterol 6 mg • Dietary Fiber 1 Gm • Sodium 203 mg • Calcium 37 mg

# Spinach-Stuffed Baked Potatoes with Goat Cheese

2 large baking potatoes (about 1 pound)

1 package (10 ounces) frozen chopped spinach, thawed, drained, and squeezed

¼ cup nonfat cottage cheese

2 ounces goat cheese with garlic and herbs

2 tablespoons chopped scallions

½ teaspoon salt

¼ teaspoon freshly ground pepper

1 tablespoon olive oil

1. Preheat the oven to 400°.

2. Scrub the potatoes and prick them several times with a fork. Bake 1 hour or until the potatoes are tender. Cool slightly.

3. Combine the spinach, cheeses, scallions, salt, and pepper in a medium bowl and set aside.

4. Cut the potatoes in half lengthwise, and carefully scoop out the pulp, leaving ¼-inch-thick shells. Mash the pulp in a small bowl until smooth and add to the spinach mixture.

5. Mound the spinach mixture into the potato shells and place them in a 9-inch square baking pan; drizzle the potatoes with oil. Bake about 15 minutes or until heated through. Serve immediately.

SERVES 2

Kilocalories 376 Kc • Protein 18 Gm • Fat 13 Gm • Percent of calories from fat 30% • Cholesterol 15 mg • Dietary Fiber 8 Gm • Sodium 908 mg • Calcium 282 mg

# Yogurt Chicken Steamed in Collards

*After the collards are steamed and the chicken is placed in the center of the leaf, it may be necessary to cut a little more of the stem end off in order to fold the leaves over the chicken.*

4 large collard leaves, stems removed
½ cup plain low-fat yogurt
1 tablespoon grainy mustard
¼ teaspoon salt
¼ cup plain dried bread crumbs

1 tablespoon toasted sesame seeds
4 boneless, skinless chicken breast halves (about 1¼ pounds)
½ cup sliced scallions

1. Rinse the collards and place them in a large nonstick skillet with ¼ cup water. Cover and cook over low heat about 10 minutes until wilted.

2. Combine the yogurt, mustard, and salt in a shallow bowl.

3. Combine the bread crumbs and sesame seeds on wax paper.

4. Dip the chicken in the yogurt mixture and coat with the bread crumb mixture. Place each breast in the center of an open collard leaf; top with the scallions. Fold one end over the chicken then fold over the other end. Place seam-side down in a collapsible steamer basket set over simmering water in a wide saucepan. Cover and steam 18 to 20 minutes or until the chicken is cooked through. Serve immediately.

SERVES 4

Kilocalories 386 Kc • Protein 49 Gm • Fat 14 Gm • Percent of calories from fat 34% • Cholesterol 120 mg • Dietary Fiber 3 Gm • Sodium 379 mg • Calcium 278 mg

# Cod and Escarole Stew

2 teaspoons vegetable oil
1 (8-ounce) cod fillet
1 garlic clove, minced
1 can (14 ounces) stewed
 tomatoes
1 cup (packed) trimmed
 escarole

½ cup wax beans (fresh, frozen,
 or canned)
2 teaspoons fresh lemon juice
¼ teaspoon dried oregano
⅛ teaspoon salt

1. Heat the oil in a medium skillet over medium heat. Add the cod and cook 2 minutes on each side. Remove from the skillet and cool slightly.

2. Add the garlic to the skillet and cook 30 seconds. Add the tomatoes, escarole, beans, juice, oregano, and salt, cover, and cook 5 minutes.

3. While the stew is cooking, on a cutting board, cut the cod into 1-inch chunks. Add to the skillet. Reduce the heat and simmer, covered, 10 minutes until the cod is cooked.

SERVES 2

Kilocalories 220 Kc • Protein 23 Gm • Fat 5 Gm • Percent of calories from fat 22% • Cholesterol 49 mg • Dietary Fiber 4 Gm • Sodium 636 mg • Calcium 118 mg

# Quail and Bitter Greens

*A romantic dinner for two.*

3 cups mixed bitter greens (arugula, dandelion, chicory, radicchio)
1 medium tomato, cut into thin wedges
¼ cup thinly sliced red onion

1 tablespoon extra-virgin olive oil
1 tablespoon raspberry vinegar
¼ teaspoon salt
⅛ teaspoon freshly ground pepper
2 quails (about 4 ounces each)

1. Preheat the broiler.

2. Combine the greens, tomato, and onion in a medium bowl.

3. Whisk the oil, vinegar, salt, and pepper with 2 tablespoons water in a 1-cup measure. Pour over the salad and toss.

4. Cut each quail in half with a sharp scissors. Coat the broiler rack with vegetable oil spray and place the quail, skin side down, on the rack in a pan 2 inches from the heat. Broil 4 minutes; turn and cook 1 minute longer, until browned.

5. Arrange the salad on 2 serving plates. Place 1 quail on each plate and serve immediately.

SERVES 2

**Variation:** Quail on Sautéed Bitter Greens: Heat 1 tablespoon oil in a medium nonstick skillet over high heat. Add 1 tablespoon chopped shallot and sauté 20 seconds. Add 4 cups mixed greens and the red onion (omit the tomato) to the skillet and sauté about 3 minutes, stirring frequently, until the greens are wilted and tender. Season with salt and pepper. Top with the broiled quail and thin slices of raw red onion.

**Kilocalories 264 Kc • Protein 19 Gm • Fat 18 Gm • Percent of calories from fat 59% • Cholesterol 65 mg • Dietary Fiber 2 Gm • Sodium 370 mg • Calcium 91 mg**

# Chicken Breasts with Watercress Sauce (Microwave)

*A cherry tomato salad is a good accompaniment to this meal, serve at room temperature.*

1 boneless, skinless chicken breast (about 1 pound) split or cut in half
¼ teaspoon salt

*Sauce:*

½ cup packed watercress, plus additional sprigs for garnish

¼ cup plain low-fat yogurt
¼ cup nonfat sour cream
1 tablespoon fresh flat-leaf parsley leaves
1 scallion (white part only)
¼ teaspoon salt
¼ teaspoon freshly ground pepper

1. Place the chicken in a glass pie plate or other microwave-safe dish.* Sprinkle with salt and cover the dish with plastic wrap. Microwave on High for 3 minutes, turning the dish a quarter turn twice (if your microwave doesn't have a turntable). Let the dish stand covered for 2 minutes. Remove the plastic and let it cool to room temperature, about 20 minutes, moistening occasionally with the juices in the dish.

2. Combine all of the sauce ingredients in a food processor fitted with the steel blade, with 1 tablespoon of juice from the chicken. Process until smooth.

3. Place the chicken breasts on serving plates; spoon the sauce over each. Garnish with watercress and serve.

SERVES 2

*Stovetop Method: To poach the chicken breasts, place them in a pan with salt and water to cover. Gently simmer, partially covered, for 20 minutes or until the chicken is no longer pink in the center.

Kilocalories 431 Kc • Protein 74 Gm • Fat 9 Gm • Percent of calories from fat 19% • Cholesterol 194 mg • Dietary Fiber 0 Gm • Sodium 799 mg • Calcium 142 mg

# 4
# Side Dishes

Side dishes used to play a supporting role on the dinner plate. Not any more. The former leading players, meat, fish, and poultry are near the top of the food pyramid and are recommended in moderate amounts. We're encouraged to choose over fifty percent of our food intake from the grains, vegetables, and fruit categories of the pyramid. To maintain a healthy balance, we should give side dishes an equal showing, if not a prominent place, at the dinner table.

A side of fries, although still appealing on occasion, has little to do with this chapter. The sides you'll find here are nutrition-smart, with the emphasis on fresh and tasty recipes that are high in flavor and imagination and low in fat and fuss. By the way, it's easy to turn these sides into vegetarian meals. Add your favorite grains and legumes to the greens to make a complete lunch or dinner.

# Kohlrabi and Mint Puree

*I had never eaten kohlrabi until I tested recipes for this book. It's been a delightful and nutritious awakening. This puree is a good substitute for mashed potatoes. In fact, you could combine this recipe with mashed potatoes for a heartier side dish.*

1 bunch kohlrabi with leaves
  (about 2¼ pounds)
1 tablespoon vegetable oil
½ cup chopped onion
¼ cup chopped fresh mint

3 tablespoons vegetable broth
1 tablespoon fresh lemon juice
1 teaspoon salt
½ teaspoon freshly ground
  pepper

1. Trim and peel the kohlrabi bulbs, reserving the leaves. Rinse and drain the leaves and coarsely chop them. Cut the bulbs into 1-inch pieces.

2. Add the bulb pieces to a pot of boiling salted water. Reduce the heat and simmer until they are tender when pierced with a fork, about 15 minutes. Add the kohlrabi leaves during the last 5 minutes of cooking.

3. Drain the kohlrabi and leaves; place in the bowl of a food processor. Add the remaining ingredients and puree until smooth.

4. Return the puree to the pot. Place over low heat, and stir until heated through, about 2 minutes. Serve immediately.

SERVES 6

Kilocalories 70 Kc • Protein 2 Gm • Fat 2 Gm • Percent of calories from fat 29% • Cholesterol 0 mg • Dietary Fiber 2 Gm • Sodium 435 mg • Calcium 49 mg

# Brussels Sprouts with Peanut Sauce

*Jazz up your Thanksgiving dinner with this unusual side dish.*

10 ounces fresh brussels sprouts, trimmed (about 3 cups)
1 teaspoon vegetable oil
2 teaspoons minced fresh ginger
1 teaspoon minced seeded jalapeño pepper
1 teaspoon ground cumin
2 tablespoons rice vinegar
2 tablespoons peanut butter
1 tablespoon fresh lemon juice
2 teaspoons sugar
1 tablespoon chopped fresh cilantro
Chopped peanuts for garnish, optional

1. Cook the brussels sprouts in boiling salted water to cover, about 10 minutes, until tender. Drain, cool slightly, and halve.

2. Heat the oil in a medium nonstick skillet over low heat. Add the ginger, jalapeño, and cumin. Cook 3 minutes, stirring occasionally.

3. Meanwhile, whisk the vinegar, peanut butter, lemon juice, sugar, and cilantro and ¼ cup water together in a 1-cup measure. Add to the skillet. Increase the heat to medium and cook 2 minutes, stirring frequently, until slightly reduced. Add the brussels sprouts and cook 2 minutes longer until heated through. Sprinkle with the peanuts, if desired, and serve immediately.

SERVES 4

Kilocalories 121 Kc • Protein 5 Gm • Fat 6 Gm • Percent of calories from fat 39% • Cholesterol 0 mg • Dietary Fiber 6 Gm • Sodium 169 mg • Calcium 53 mg

# Braised Collards with Potatoes and Red Pepper Oil

*To make your own red pepper oil, heat 1 tablespoon olive oil over medium heat in a small skillet. Add ¼ teaspoon red pepper flakes and cook about 30 seconds, until sizzling.*

1 bunch collard greens (about 1½ pounds), trimmed and coarsely chopped

1 pound small new potatoes, quartered

½ teaspoon salt

1 tablespoon red pepper oil

2 large garlic cloves, thinly sliced

1. Combine the collards and potatoes in a deep skillet. Add about 1 cup water (or enough to just cover the vegetables) and the salt. Cover tightly and bring to a boil. Reduce the heat to medium and cook, covered, about 15 minutes or until the potatoes are tender. Uncover, turn the heat to high, and cook until the water is evaporated.

2. While the collards are cooking, heat the oil over low heat in a small skillet. Add the garlic slices and cook until they are just lightly browned, about 3 minutes. Pour over the vegetables and stir to combine. Serve immediately.

SERVES 4

Kilocalories 161 Kc • Protein 4 Gm • Fat 4 Gm • Percent of calories from fat 20% • Cholesterol 0 mg • Dietary Fiber 2 Gm • Sodium 321 mg • Calcium 45 mg

# Dandelion with Lemon and Olive Oil

4 cups coarsely chopped
dandelion greens
1 teaspoon grated lemon zest

2 tablespoons fresh lemon
juice
1 tablespoon olive oil
Coarse salt

Steam the dandelion greens 15 minutes. Place in a serving bowl and combine with the lemon zest, juice, and oil. Sprinkle with salt and serve.

SERVES 4

Kilocalories 59 Kc • Protein 2 Gm • Fat 4 Gm • Percent of calories from fat 53%
• Cholesterol 0 mg • Dietary Fiber 3 Gm • Sodium 36 mg • Calcium 114 mg

# Savory Bread Pudding with Turnip Greens

1 package (16 ounces) frozen turnip greens, thawed, drained, and squeezed
4 cups 1-inch cubes day-old Italian bread
2 cups skim milk
2 large eggs

3 tablespoons grated Romano cheese
1 tablespoon chopped fresh savory (1 teaspoon dried)
½ teaspoon salt
¼ teaspoon garlic powder
¼ teaspoon ground red pepper

1. Preheat the oven to 375°.

2. Combine the greens and bread in a 1½-quart casserole.

3. Whisk the milk, eggs, cheese, and spices together in a 4-cup measure. Pour over the greens mixture, saturating the bread.

4. Place the casserole dish in a slightly larger baking pan. Pour hot water into the pan to reach halfway up the sides of the dish. Bake 45 to 50 minutes until just set. Carefully remove the casserole from the pan and cool 10 minutes.

SERVES 4

Kilocalories 259 Kc • Protein 17 Gm • Fat 6 Gm • Percent of calories from fat 21% • Cholesterol 113 mg • Dietary Fiber 1 Gm • Sodium 729 mg • Calcium 425 mg

# Gingered Red Cabbage and Pineapple

*The acid from the pineapple juice turns the cabbage into neon purple. Your kids will love it.*

1 package (18 ounces) peeled
  and cored fresh pineapple
2 teaspoons vegetable oil

1 tablespoon minced fresh ginger
4 cups shredded red cabbage
¼ teaspoon salt

1. Reserve ½ cup pineapple juice. Cut the pineapple into 1-inch chunks (about 2 cups). Set aside.

2. Heat the oil in a large nonstick skillet over medium heat; add the ginger and cook 30 seconds. Stir in the cabbage. Add the reserved juice and cook 10 minutes, stirring occasionally. Add the pineapple and cook 2 minutes longer, until heated through.

SERVES 4

Kilocalories 108 Kc • Protein 2 Gm • Fat 3 Gm • Percent of calories from fat 23% • Cholesterol 0 mg • Dietary Fiber 3 Gm • Sodium 156 mg • Calcium 53 mg

# Grilled Endive with Mustard Vinaigrette (Outdoor Grill)

*Mustard vinaigrette is actually "the" classic French dressing, bearing no resemblance to the bottled version.*

1 tablespoon olive oil
1 teaspoon red wine vinegar
½ teaspoon chopped fresh chervil (or marjoram)
¼ teaspoon dry mustard

¼ teaspoon salt
¼ teaspoon Worcestershire sauce
4 medium heads Belgian endive, trimmed and halved lengthwise

1. Coat your grill rack with vegetable oil spray; place 5 inches from the coals or heat source.

2. To prepare the dressing, combine the oil, vinegar, chervil, mustard, salt, and Worcestershire sauce with 2 tablespoons water in a small saucepan. Place the pan on the grill; bring it to a simmer. Brush the cut sides of the endive with the dressing and grill over medium-hot coals 5 minutes. Turn and brush with the remaining dressing. Grill 4 minutes until barely tender.

3. Arrange the endive on a serving platter and drizzle with the remaining dressing. Serve hot or at room temperature.

SERVES 4

Kilocalories 48 Kc • Protein 1 Gm • Fat 3 Gm • Percent of calories from fat 62% • Cholesterol 0 mg • Dietary Fiber 3 Gm • Sodium 165 mg • Calcium 21 mg

# Brussels Sprouts and Mandarin Oranges

*Brussels sprouts are the most perfect miniature head of leafy greens found on the planet.*

2 cups trimmed fresh brussels sprouts, halved, or 1 package (10 ounces) frozen, thawed
1 tablespoon unsalted butter
1 teaspoon crushed, toasted cumin seed
1 teaspoon mustard seed
¼ teaspoon salt
¼ teaspoon freshly ground pepper
½ cup coarsely chopped onion
1 garlic clove, minced
2 large mandarin oranges, peeled and segmented, or 1 can (11 ounces) mandarin segments, drained

1. Pour ½ cup water into a medium saucepan; bring to a boil. Add the brussels sprouts and cook 5 minutes, separating the sprouts, if they're still a bit frozen, with a wooden spoon. Drain.

2. Melt the butter in a large nonstick skillet over high heat. Stir in the cumin, mustard seed, salt, and pepper. Add the brussels sprouts, onion, and garlic and cook 2 to 3 minutes, stirring frequently, until lightly browned. Add the orange segments and cook 1 minute longer, stirring. Serve immediately.

SERVES 4

Kilocalories 107 Kc • Protein 3 Gm • Fat 4 Gm • Percent of calories from fat 31% • Cholesterol 8 mg • Dietary Fiber 4 Gm • Sodium 166 mg • Calcium 58 mg

# Spinach Siciliana

1 tablespoon olive oil
1½ pounds fresh spinach,
    trimmed and coarsely chopped
    (wet)
¼ cup raisins

1 tablespoon pignoli nuts,
    toasted
2 teaspoons unsalted
    butter
¼ teaspoon salt

1. Heat the oil in a large nonstick skillet or saucepan over medium heat; remove the pan from the heat. Carefully add the wet spinach. Cover and cook 5 to 10 minutes until the spinach is wilted, stirring occasionally.

2. Stir in the raisins, nuts, butter, and salt. Cover and cook 3 to 5 minutes longer. Serve immediately.

SERVES 4

Kilocalories 125 Kc • Protein 6 Gm • Fat 7 Gm • Percent of calories from fat 46% • Cholesterol 5 mg • Dietary Fiber 5 Gm • Sodium 281 mg • Calcium 174 mg

# Smothered Broccoli Raab

*Broccoli raab "affogata" is an old Italian method for cooking greens.*

1 tablespoon olive oil
4 large garlic cloves, crushed
½ teaspoon red pepper flakes

1½ pounds broccoli raab,
    trimmed and coarsely chopped
½ teaspoon coarse salt

1. Heat the oil in a large saucepan over medium heat; add the garlic and pepper. Cook about 3 minutes until the garlic is golden.

2. Carefully add the greens and salt to the pot; cover and cook 25 minutes. Serve immediately.

SERVES 4

**Variation:** Substitute spinach for the broccoli raab and add ⅛ teaspoon grated nutmeg.

Kilocalories 69 Kc • Protein 2 Gm • Fat 4 Gm • Percent of calories from fat 45% • Cholesterol 0 mg • Dietary Fiber 5 Gm • Sodium 341 mg • Calcium 239 mg

# Arugula and Marmalade Sweet Potatoes

2 cups (packed) chopped arugula
¼ cup chicken broth
¼ teaspoon Chinese five-spice powder

1 large sweet potato (about 1 pound)
¼ cup orange marmalade

1. Preheat the oven to 350°. Place the arugula in the bottom of an 11 × 7-inch baking pan coated with vegetable oil spray. Add the broth and sprinkle with the spice.

2. Trim off the ends of the potato and cut the potato into ½-inch rounds. Arrange the rounds in a single layer on top of the arugula and brush with the marmalade. Cover tightly with foil and bake 45 minutes. Uncover, increase the temperature to 400°, and bake 15 minutes until some of the liquid is absorbed.

SERVES 4

Kilocalories 173 Kc • Protein 2 Gm • Fat 0 Gm • Percent of calories from fat 2% • Cholesterol 0 mg • Dietary Fiber 4 Gm • Sodium 23 mg • Calcium 55 mg

# Cabbage and Onion Compote

*Slow cooking heightens the sweetness of this chilled dish. It's delicious with grilled chicken or fish and will keep in the refrigerator for up to 2 weeks.*

1 tablespoon vegetable oil
2 cups shredded cabbage
2 cups thinly sliced onion
½ cup red wine vinegar

2 tablespoons honey
½ teaspoon salt
⅛ teaspoon ground
  cinnamon

1. Heat the oil in a 3-quart saucepan over medium-high heat; add the cabbage and onion. Cook about 15 minutes until the onion starts to brown, stirring frequently.

2. Stir in the vinegar, scraping the bottom of the pot to loosen bits and pieces. Add the honey and cook until the vinegar evaporates, then add ¼ cup of water. Reduce the heat and simmer, uncovered, stirring frequently, until the liquid has been absorbed and the mixture is lightly browned, about 10 minutes.

3. Remove from the heat and season with the salt and cinnamon. Cool completely and refrigerate until ready to use.

SERVES 4

Kilocalories 136 Kc • Protein 1 Gm • Fat 4 Gm • Percent of calories from fat 29% • Cholesterol 0 mg • Dietary Fiber 2 Gm • Sodium 306 mg • Calcium 42 mg

# Tat Soi and Jerusalem Artichoke Stir-Fry

*Tat soi is a Japanese mustard green, with shiny green leaves and peppery flavor. Serve with jasmine or basmati rice for a delicious vegetarian meal.*

1 cup (about 5 ounces) small Jerusalem artichokes, peeled and sliced ⅛ inch thick (drained canned water chestnuts may be substituted)

1 tablespoon low-sodium soy sauce

2 teaspoons dark sesame oil

2 teaspoons minced fresh ginger

2 medium garlic cloves, minced

8 cups coarsely chopped tat soi

2 tablespoons toasted sesame seeds, optional

1. Combine the artichokes and soy sauce in a small bowl; let them stand for 10 minutes.

2. Heat a wok or deep skillet over high heat. Add the oil and swirl around until sizzling. Add the ginger and garlic and cook 20 to 30 seconds until barely browned.

3. Stir in the tat soi and the artichoke mixture. Cook 3 minutes until the artichokes are tender, stirring constantly. Sprinkle with sesame seeds, if desired.

SERVES 3

Kilocalories 88 Kc • Protein 4 Gm • Fat 3 Gm • Percent of calories from fat 32% • Cholesterol 0 mg • Dietary Fiber 1 Gm • Sodium 242 mg • Calcium 116 mg

# Braised Endive, Fennel, and Tomato

2 heads Belgian endive
2 teaspoons olive oil
2 large garlic cloves
2 medium fennel bulbs, halved
   lengthwise

1 cup vegetable broth
¼ teaspoon salt
¼ teaspoon freshly ground
   pepper
1 medium tomato, chopped

1. Preheat the oven to 400°.

2. Trim the ends from the endive and cut in half lengthwise.

3. Heat the oil in a large ovenproof skillet over low heat. Add the garlic and cook 5 minutes or until lightly browned. Remove the garlic with a slotted spoon and set it aside.

4. Increase the heat to medium. Place the fennel halves, cut sides down, in the skillet and cook for 5 minutes. Add the endive halves, cut sides down, and cook 3 minutes longer or until browned.

5. Add the broth, salt, and pepper and stir to loosen bits and pieces from the bottom of the skillet. Top with the tomato, cover, and bake for 30 minutes, until tender. Garnish with the reserved garlic.

SERVES 4

Kilocalories 59 Kc • Protein 2 Gm • Fat 2 Gm • Percent of calories from fat 34%
• Cholesterol 0 mg • Dietary Fiber 2 Gm • Sodium 193 mg • Calcium 35 mg

# Sautéed Collards with Spicy Yogurt

*This dish is adapted from a recipe by my favorite Southern cookbook author, Sarah Belk.*

⅓ cup plain nonfat yogurt
1 tablespoon Dijon mustard
1 pound fresh collard greens,
    trimmed

1 tablespoon vegetable oil
½ cup diced onion
½ teaspoon salt

1. Combine the yogurt and mustard and set aside.

2. Stack and cut the collards in 1-inch strips, then chop. Add the greens to a large pot of boiling salted water. Cook 10 minutes or until just tender. Drain.

3. Heat the oil in large nonstick skillet over medium heat. Add the onion, cover, and cook 2 to 3 minutes, until soft. Stir in the greens and salt. Reduce the heat and stir in the yogurt mixture. Cook about 5 minutes or until the liquid evaporates. Serve immediately.

SERVES 3

**Variation:** For a delicious bruschetta appetizer for six, grill ½-inch-thick slices of Tuscan bread (round, peasant-style Italian bread) until lightly browned. Rub with cut slices of garlic and top with the prepared collard greens and a dash of black pepper.

Kilocalories 105 Kc • Protein 4 Gm • Fat 5 Gm • Percent of calories from fat 42%
• Cholesterol 1 mg • Dietary Fiber 1 Gm • Sodium 457 mg • Calcium 92 mg

# Braised Chinese Cabbage
# with Green Beans and Onions

2 teaspoons vegetable oil
½ cup diced onion
½ cup sliced scallions
4 cups chopped Chinese or napa
   cabbage

2 cups trimmed green beans
   (8 ounces), cut into 1-inch
   pieces
2 cups canned vegetable juice
¼ teaspoon salt

1. Heat the oil in a Dutch oven over medium heat. Add the onion and scallions and cook 3 minutes, stirring frequently, until softened.

2. Add the cabbage, green beans, and juice. Bring to a boil; reduce the heat and simmer, uncovered, 45 minutes, stirring occasionally. Season with the salt.

SERVES 4

Kilocalories 94 Kc • Protein 3 Gm • Fat 3 Gm • Percent of calories from fat 24% • Cholesterol 0 mg • Dietary Fiber 5 Gm • Sodium 604 mg • Calcium 88 mg

# Cabbage, Olives, and Capers

*This makes a wonderful main dish meal when mixed with pasta. Just toss the pasta with 1 to 2 tablespoons olive oil, then stir into the cabbage mixture. Serve with garlic bread.*

8 cups savoy cabbage (about 1½ pounds)
3 teaspoons olive oil
2 teaspoons sugar
1 cup chicken or vegetable broth
1 tablespoon rinsed capers

8 kalamata olives, pitted and chopped
¼ teaspoon salt
¼ teaspoon freshly ground pepper

1. Combine the cabbage, 2 teaspoons of the oil, and the sugar in a large nonstick skillet. Cover and cook over low heat for 15 minutes, stirring occasionally.

2. Increase the heat to medium and add the broth, capers, olives, salt, and pepper. Cook, uncovered, 10 to 15 minutes until the cabbage is browned and the liquid is evaporated, stirring frequently. To serve, drizzle with the remaining 1 teaspoon oil.

SERVES 4

Kilocalories 96 Kc • Protein 4 Gm • Fat 5 Gm • Percent of calories from fat 43% • Cholesterol 1 mg • Dietary Fiber 4 Gm • Sodium 363 mg • Calcium 57 mg

# Steamed Broccoli Raab
# with Garlic Butter

1 tablespoon unsalted butter
1 small garlic clove
¼ teaspoon lemon pepper

1 bunch broccoli raab (about 1¼
  pounds), trimmed and chopped

1. Combine the butter, garlic, and lemon pepper in a small food processor. Process until smooth.

2. Place the broccoli raab in a collapsible vegetable steamer set over simmering water in a wide saucepan. Cover and steam 5 to 7 minutes until tender. Place the broccoli raab in a serving bowl and toss with the garlic butter. Serve immediately.

SERVES 4

Kilocalories 57 Kc • Protein 2 Gm • Fat 3 Gm • Percent of calories from fat 48%
• Cholesterol 8 mg • Dietary Fiber 4 Gm • Sodium 42 mg • Calcium 197 mg

# Braised Red Cabbage

2 tablespoons olive oil
½ cup chopped onion
6 cups finely shredded red
   cabbage (about
   1¼ pounds)
2 cups red wine or water

3 whole cloves tied in
   cheesecloth
2 teaspoons sugar
¼ teaspoon salt
⅛ teaspoon freshly ground
   pepper

1. Heat the oil in a large saucepan over medium-high heat. Add the onion and cook for 2 minutes until softened, stirring frequently.

2. Reduce the heat; add the cabbage, wine, cloves, and sugar. Simmer, covered, for about 1 hour until tender, adding more liquid if necessary. Remove from the heat and discard the cheesecloth. Season with the salt and pepper. Serve immediately.

SERVES 4

Kilocalories 199 Kc • Protein 2 Gm • Fat 7 Gm • Percent of calories from fat 31% • Cholesterol 0 mg • Dietary Fiber 2 Gm • Sodium 169 mg • Calcium 67 mg

# Wilted Spinach with Clementines

*Clementines, part of the mandarin orange family, look like tiny tangerines. In fact, they are a cross between tangerines and Seville oranges. Pere Clement, a French priest, cultivated this fruit at the turn of the century in Algeria.*

1 teaspoon vegetable oil
¼ cup minced red onion
1 package (10 ounces) fresh
    spinach, washed and trimmed
⅛ teaspoon salt

⅛ teaspoon ground cinnamon
2 clementine tangerines, peeled
    and segments separated, or
    1 seedless orange, cut in thin
    slices

1. Heat the oil in a medium saucepan over medium heat. Add the onion and cook 2 to 3 minutes, until softened.

2. Stir in the spinach, cover, and cook about 2 minutes until the spinach wilts. Season with the salt and cinnamon. Remove from the heat and stir in the clementines. Serve immediately.

SERVES 2

Kilocalories 96 Kc • Protein 5 Gm • Fat 3 Gm • Percent of calories from fat 24% • Cholesterol 0 mg • Dietary Fiber 6 Gm • Sodium 259 mg • Calcium 158 mg

# Chinese Cabbage, Watercress, and Carrot Slaw

*A creamy, sweet slaw with fennel overtones.*

2 cups shredded Chinese
   cabbage
2 cups shredded carrot
1 cup (packed) chopped
   watercress

*Dressing:*

½ cup reduced-calorie
   mayonnaise
¼ cup 1% milk
2 tablespoons fresh lemon juice
1 tablespoon honey
½ teaspoon crushed fennel seeds
¼ teaspoon salt

1. Combine the cabbage, carrot, and watercress in a serving bowl.

2. Whisk all of the dressing ingredients together until blended. Pour the dressing over the slaw and toss. Refrigerate, covered, until ready to serve.

SERVES 4

Kilocalories 133 Kc • Protein 2 Gm • Fat 6 Gm • Percent of calories from fat 41% • Cholesterol 8 mg • Dietary Fiber 3 Gm • Sodium 345 mg • Calcium 60 mg

# New Potatoes and Dandelion

*A peasant-style, coarsely mashed potato dish. Once you try olive oil in potatoes, you may never use butter again.*

2 pounds tiny new potatoes, washed and scrubbed
4 cups coarsely chopped dandelion greens
¼ cup extra-virgin olive oil

¼ cup chopped fresh basil
1 teaspoon salt
½ teaspoon freshly ground pepper

1. Place the potatoes in a large pot of boiling, salted water. Reduce the heat to medium high. Cover and cook 15 minutes. Add the dandelion and cook 5 to 10 minutes longer or until the potatoes are tender when pierced with a fork. Drain.

2. Mash the potatoes in the pot. Stir in the oil, basil, salt, and pepper. Serve immediately.

SERVES 6

Kilocalories 217 Kc • Protein 4 Gm • Fat 9 Gm • Percent of calories from fat 37% • Cholesterol 0 mg • Dietary Fiber 4 Gm • Sodium 420 mg • Calcium 89 mg

# Blanched Escarole and Fried Capers

*A zester is a handy tool to have for making very thin strips from the outer colored layer of lemons, oranges, or grapefruit and a definite plus to have on hand for this recipe.*

1 bunch escarole (about 1 pound), trimmed and shredded
1 tablespoon extra-virgin olive oil
1 tablespoon unsalted capers, drained

½ teaspoon salt
Freshly ground pepper
2 teaspoons thinly sliced lemon zest for garnish, optional

1. Drop the escarole in a pot of salted boiling water. Cook 3 to 5 minutes until it is as tender as you like. Drain well.

2. While the escarole is cooking, heat the oil in a large nonstick skillet over medium heat. Add the capers and cook 2 minutes; remove with a slotted spoon.

3. Stir in the drained escarole, salt, and pepper and heat through. Place on a serving plate and top with the capers and lemon zest, if using. Serve immediately.

SERVES 4

Kilocalories 49 Kc • Protein 1 Gm • Fat 4 Gm • Percent of calories from fat 60% • Cholesterol 0 mg • Dietary Fiber 4 Gm • Sodium 316 mg • Calcium 59 mg

# Rhubarb and Spinach Compote

*Rhubarb and spinach—harbingers of spring—are combined in this tasty chilled dish. Try it instead of relish.*

1 cup apple cider vinegar
⅓ cup (packed) dark brown sugar
4 cups chopped trimmed rhubarb
4 cups chopped fresh spinach

½ cup chopped onion
¼ teaspoon salt
½ teaspoon ground allspice

1. Combine the vinegar and sugar with 1 cup water in a Dutch oven. Bring to a boil, stirring occasionally, until the sugar is dissolved.

2. Reduce the heat and stir in the rhubarb, spinach, onion, salt, and all-spice. Cover and simmer 30 minutes, stirring occasionally. Uncover, turn the heat to high, and cook, stirring frequently, until thick and syrupy, about 15 minutes. Cool, cover, and refrigerate up to 1 week.

MAKES 6 (1/3 CUP EACH)

Kilocalories 82 Kc • Protein 2 Gm • Fat 0 Gm • Percent of calories from fat 3% • Cholesterol 0 mg • Dietary Fiber 3 Gm • Sodium 135 mg • Calcium 123 mg

# Stuffed Escarole
# (Pressure Cooker and Stovetop)

*These escarole wedges look beautiful on an antipasto platter which might also include roasted red peppers, olives, and fennel. This recipe may be halved.*

½ cup raisins
2 medium heads escarole (about 2½ pounds)
1½ tablespoons olive oil
8 garlic cloves, minced
¼ teaspoon red pepper flakes
1 cup plain dried bread crumbs

¼ cup chopped pignoli nuts
¼ cup chopped Italian green olives (about 4 large)
¼ cup grated Romano cheese
¼ teaspoon salt
1 cup vegetable broth or water

1. Soak the raisins in hot water to cover for 15 minutes. Drain.

2. Rinse the whole escarole heads to remove grit and dirt. Drain.

3. Heat ½ tablespoon of the oil in an open pressure cooker* over medium heat. Add the garlic and red pepper flakes and cook 30 seconds. Lower the heat; stir in the bread crumbs and nuts. Cook 3 to 4 minutes until the bread crumbs brown, stirring frequently. Remove from the heat and combine the bread crumb mixture with the raisins, olives, cheese, and salt in a medium bowl.

4. Pour the vegetable broth into the cooker; place steamer rack on top.

5. Carefully open the escarole leaves, leaving them attached to the core. Spoon half of the filling between the leaves. Close the leaves and tie with a string to secure. Repeat the procedure with the remaining head of escarole. Place in the cooker and lock the lid in place. Bring to full pressure over high heat. Adjust the heat to maintain high pressure and cook for 5 minutes. Release the pressure by placing the edge of the pot under running cold water. Remove the lid, tilting it away from you to allow excess steam to escape.

6. Carefully lift out the escarole with flexible spatulas. Place on a large cutting board and let them stand for 10 minutes. Remove the string and cut the escarole lengthwise into 4 wedges; repeat with the remaining escarole. Place on a serving platter. These may be served hot or at room temperature with a light drizzle of extra-virgin olive oil.

SERVES 8

**Variation:** Use dried chopped figs instead of raisins. Eliminate the cheese and use flavored or whole wheat bread crumbs.

*Stovetop Method: Increase the broth to 2 cups. Step 3: Heat the oil in a deep skillet and follow the remaining instruction for that step. Pour the broth into the skillet and set aside. Stuff the escarole as in step 5 and place in the broth. Bring to a simmer, cover, and cook until the escarole is tender, 30 to 40 minutes. Let it stand 10 minutes, remove the string, and slice.

Kilocalories 179 Kc • Protein 6 Gm • Fat 8 Gm • Percent of calories from fat 35% • Cholesterol 3 mg • Dietary Fiber 6 Gm • Sodium 353 mg • Calcium 149 mg

# Chicken Sausage–Stuffed Tomatoes

4 large beefsteak tomatoes
½ teaspoon salt
1½ tablespoons olive oil
1 small onion, finely chopped
1 garlic clove, minced
¼ teaspoon fennel seeds
¼ teaspoon red pepper flakes

¼ pound (bulk) chicken or
  meatless sausage
½ cup finely chopped cooked
  spinach
½ cup plain dried bread crumbs
2 cups Bibb lettuce for garnish,
  optional

1. Preheat the oven to 350°.

2. Wash and dry the tomatoes. Cut off the tops with a serrated knife; scoop out the pulp, leaving only the shell; reserve the pulp.

3. Sprinkle the inside of each shell evenly with the salt; place upside down on paper towels to drain for 30 minutes.

4. Heat 1 tablespoon of the oil in a small nonstick skillet over medium heat; add the onion, garlic, fennel seed, and red pepper flakes; cook 5 minutes. Add the sausage and cook until no longer pink, about 5 minutes. Stir in the reserved tomato pulp and spinach and cook 1 minute. Remove from the heat and stir in the bread crumbs.

5. Fill each tomato with the sausage mixture. Place the stuffed tomatoes in an 8-inch square pan. Drizzle with the remaining ½ tablespoon oil. Bake 20 to 30 minutes until the top is lightly browned; remove with a slotted spoon and place on a bed of lettuce, if desired.

SERVES 4

Kilocalories 205 Kc • Protein 9 Gm • Fat 9 Gm • Percent of calories from fat 38% • Cholesterol 15 mg • Dietary Fiber 3 Gm • Sodium 705 mg • Calcium 108 mg

# Spinach and "Bacon" (Microwave)

*This recipe calls for soy bacon bits, but if you're energetic, cook up a slice of turkey or meatless bacon and dice it.*

1 cup finely chopped onion
1 tablespoon vegetable oil
8 cups spinach leaves, coarsely
   chopped (wet)

1 tablespoon soy bacon bits
½ teaspoon salt

1. Combine the onion and oil in a 2-quart microwave-safe bowl. Cover and microwave on High for 2 to 3 minutes, until the onion is tender.

2. Add the wet spinach, bacon bits, and salt. Cover and microwave on High for about 6 minutes, until the spinach is wilted. Let it stand for 3 minutes; stir well and serve.

SERVES 4

Kilocalories 77 Kc • Protein 4 Gm • Fat 5 Gm • Percent of calories from fat 47%
• Cholesterol 0 mg • Dietary Fiber 4 Gm • Sodium 413 mg • Calcium 120 mg

# Braised Mixed Greens

*These greens are cooked long and slow.*

2 tablespoons peanut oil
½ cup finely chopped onion
½ cup finely chopped celery
12 cups chopped, mixed greens
   (collard, turnip, mustard, kale,
   or dandelion)

1 tablespoon apple cider vinegar
½ teaspoon red pepper flakes
½ teaspoon salt

1. Heat the oil in a Dutch oven over medium heat. Add the onion and celery; cook 5 minutes, until tender, stirring occasionally.

2. Stir in the greens. Cover and cook 10 minutes, until wilted, stirring occasionally.

3. Add the vinegar, red pepper flakes, and salt; cover and cook 5 minutes.

4. Add 2 cups water, reduce the heat, and simmer 1½ hours, adding more water if necessary.

SERVES 4

Kilocalories 122 Kc • Protein 4 Gm • Fat 8 Gm • Percent of calories from fat 51% • Cholesterol 0 mg • Dietary Fiber 5 Gm • Sodium 368 mg • Calcium 185 mg

# Red Peppers and Escarole

2 tablespoons olive oil
2 cups seeded and thinly sliced
  red bell pepper
4 cups (packed) coarsely chopped
  escarole (wet)

12 pitted olives, halved
1 tablespoon balsamic
  vinegar
¼ teaspoon salt
Freshly ground pepper

1. Heat the oil in a large nonstick skillet over high heat. Add the bell pepper and cook 1 to 2 minutes, stirring frequently, until lightly browned.

2. Stir in the wet escarole. Reduce the heat, cover, and cook about 5 minutes until wilted and tender. Uncover, add the olives, vinegar, salt, and ground pepper and cook 1 minute longer. Serve immediately.

SERVES 4

Kilocalories 118 Kc • Protein 2 Gm • Fat 8 Gm • Percent of calories from fat 60% • Cholesterol 0 mg • Dietary Fiber 3 Gm • Sodium 274 mg • Calcium 48 mg

# Spinach Timbales

*A timbale is a molded dish. In this recipe, custard cups are used.*

4½ teaspoons all-purpose flour
1½ tablespoons unsalted butter
½ cup minced onion
½ cup evaporated skimmed milk

2 large eggs, at room
 temperature, separated
2 cups (packed) finely chopped
 fresh spinach
¼ teaspoon grated nutmeg

1. Preheat the oven to 350°. Coat four 6-ounce custard cups with vegetable oil spray. Using about ½ teaspoon of the flour, dust the cups evenly, and set aside.

2. Melt the butter in a medium nonstick saucepan, over medium heat. Add the onion and cook 5 minutes, until tender. Whisk in the remaining 4 teaspoons flour and cook 1 minute, stirring constantly. Gradually pour in the milk. Continue cooking, stirring constantly, about 3 minutes, until thick.

3. Beat the egg yolks in a small bowl; stir in 2 tablespoons of the hot milk mixture. Return the yolk mixture to the saucepan and cook 30 seconds. Remove from the heat; stir in the spinach and nutmeg. Scrape into a large bowl. Cover and set aside.

4. Beat the egg whites in a small bowl, with an electric mixer on high speed, until stiff but not dry. Stir one fourth of the whites into the spinach mixture. Fold in the remaining whites until no white streaks remain. Spoon evenly into the prepared cups. Smooth the tops and place the cups on a baking sheet. Bake 15 to 20 minutes or until browned and puffy. The timbales may be served in the custard cups placed on serving dishes, or, if desired, run a knife around the rim edges of the cups and invert them onto serving plates to release the spinach mixture.

SERVES 4

Kilocalories 128 Kc • Protein 7 Gm • Fat 7 Gm • Percent of calories from fat 51%
• Cholesterol 119 mg • Dietary Fiber 1 Gm • Sodium 92 mg • Calcium 141 mg

# Vegetables in Pepper Baskets (Microwave)

4 medium yellow or red bell peppers, about 4 inches high
1 package (10 ounces) frozen chopped kale, thawed, drained, and squeezed
½ cup part-skim ricotta cheese
½ cup shredded reduced-fat Monterey Jack cheese (1½ ounces)

1½ teaspoons chopped fresh marjoram (½ teaspoon dried)
¼ teaspoon salt
8 broccoli spears, about 3½ inches long
½ cup julienne of carrots
½ cup julienne of summer squash
6 asparagus spears, trimmed and halved crosswise
½ cup trimmed green beans

1. Cut angled slices from the tops of the bell peppers, leaving a shell with a 4-inch back and 3-inch front. Remove the seeds. Discard the stem and chop the remaining pepper top.

2. Combine the kale, chopped bell pepper, cheeses, marjoram, and salt in a medium bowl. Spoon equal amounts of the mixture into each pepper. Arrange the broccoli and other vegetables upright in the peppers and place the peppers on a microwave-safe plate. For each pepper, soak 2 unseparated sheets of microwave-safe paper towels under running water; squeeze out the excess water. Fold the paper towels in half and cover each pepper, tucking the ends of the towels under. Microwave on High 8 to 10 minutes or until the peppers are tender yet firm. Remove the peppers to a double thickness of paper towels to drain any excess liquid.

Serve immediately.

SERVES 4

Kilocalories 145 Kc • Protein 12 Gm • Fat 5 Gm • Percent of calories from fat 28% • Cholesterol 18 mg • Dietary Fiber 4 Gm • Sodium 299 mg • Calcium 301 mg

# Kale Stuffing

*Although this is a side dish, there is enough stuffing for a 4-pound roasting chicken.**

1 tablespoon vegetable oil
1 cup chopped onion
1 package (10 ounces) frozen chopped kale, thawed (with juice)
1 cup plain dried bread crumbs

½ cup chicken broth
1 large egg white
1 teaspoon dried thyme, crumbled
¼ teaspoon salt
¼ teaspoon freshly ground pepper

1. Preheat the oven to 375°.
2. Heat the oil in a large nonstick skillet over low heat. Add the onion; toss to coat. Cover and cook 5 to 8 minutes until the onion is softened. Remove from the heat. Stir in the kale and the bread crumbs, broth, egg white, thyme, salt, and pepper. Mix the stuffing with your hands. Spoon into a 9-inch square baking pan coated with vegetable oil spray. Cover with foil and bake 15 to 20 minutes until heated through.

SERVES 4

*To stuff a chicken, lightly spoon the stuffing into the cavity of the chicken. Cover the cavity with foil. Place the chicken on a roasting rack in a baking pan. Roast about 2 hours in a 350° oven or until a thermometer inserted into the thickest part of the thigh registers 185°. Let it stand 10 minutes before carving.

**Variation:** Pita Sandwiches: To serve leftover stuffing, cover with foil and place in a 350° oven until heated through or microwave covered with plastic wrap. Place the stuffing in the bottom of a pita bread; top with finely shredded lettuce or cabbage. Combine yogurt, salsa, and ground cumin (to taste) and spoon into the pita.

**Kilocalories 184 Kc • Protein 7 Gm • Fat 6 Gm • Percent of calories from fat 27% • Cholesterol 1 mg • Dietary Fiber 2 Gm • Sodium 415 mg • Calcium 175 mg**

# Kale, Prune, and Apple Stuffing

16 slices reduced-calorie whole wheat bread, cut into ½-inch cubes

1 package (10 ounces) frozen chopped kale, thawed (with juice) or 1 can (14 ounces) chopped kale, drained and squeezed

1 can (13¾ ounces) vegetable broth

1 Golden Delicious apple, peeled and grated

½ cup chopped celery

8 pitted prunes, chopped

1 large whole egg

1 egg white

1 teaspoon poultry seasoning

¼ teaspoon salt

1. Preheat the oven to 375°.
2. Toast the bread cubes in the oven on a baking sheet.
3. Combine the kale, broth, apple, celery, and prunes in a large skillet. Bring to a boil over medium heat. Reduce the heat, cover, and simmer about 10 minutes until the celery is tender, stirring occasionally. Place the mixture in a large bowl. Add the egg, egg white, poultry seasoning, salt and ½ cup water to the stuffing. Mix the stuffing with your hands. Spoon the mixture into a 9-inch square baking pan coated with vegetable oil spray. Cover with foil, and bake 15 to 20 minutes.

SERVES 4

Kilocalories 354 Kc • Protein 15 Gm • Fat 4 Gm • Percent of calories from fat 10% • Cholesterol 53 mg • Dietary Fiber 14 Gm • Sodium 1089 mg • Calcium 215 mg

# 5

# Pasta Plus

Pasta literally means "dough" in Italian. In Italy there are three kinds of pasta—one for breads, one for tarts, and one for macaroni.

In my childhood home, pasta referred to a sweet dough (*pasta frolla*) used for Easter and Christmas pies. What is now commonly referred to as pasta, we simply called macaroni (maccheroni).

On Sundays we always had macaroni with a long-simmered, tomato-based meat sauce. But during the week, macaroni was tossed with greens and other vegetables, beans, cheese, and fish, and often dressed with sautéed garlic and olive oil. Those are the dishes that inspired this chapter.

"Pasta Plus" includes the pasta dishes of my youth, as well as Asian and Greek-style dishes and a uniquely American slant on the theme.

It is important to use freshly grated cheese in these pasta dishes for authentic flavor. *Buon appetito!*

# Pastina and Spinach Casserole

½ cup pastina macaroni

1 package (10 ounces) fresh spinach, trimmed and coarsely chopped

1 cup nonfat cottage cheese

¼ cup grated Romano cheese

¼ cup 1% milk

2 tablespoons seasoned dried bread crumbs

1 tablespoon chopped fresh flat-leaf parsley

⅛ teaspoon ground nutmeg

1. Preheat the oven to 350°.

2. Boil 2 cups water in a medium saucepan. Add the pastina and cook 3 minutes. Top with the spinach, push down, cover, and cook 2 minutes. Remove from the heat and stir to combine.

3. Combine the cheeses and milk with 1 tablespoon of the bread crumbs, parsley, and nutmeg in a 1½-quart casserole. Stir in the spinach mixture until blended. Top with the remaining 1 tablespoon bread crumbs. Bake for 35 minutes. Let the dish stand 5 minutes before serving.

SERVES 4

Kilocalories 158 Kc • Protein 15 Gm • Fat 3 Gm • Percent of calories from fat 14% • Cholesterol 12 mg • Dietary Fiber 2 Gm • Sodium 434 mg • Calcium 189 mg

# Greek-Style Farfalle

*This Mediterranean dish features* farfalle, *the Italian word for butterflies. On this side of the Atlantic, farfalle macaroni is often referred to as "bowties."*

1 pound farfalle pasta
3 tablespoons olive oil
1 can (15 ounces) chickpeas, drained
3 large garlic cloves, minced
½ cup chicken broth
½ teaspoon dried oregano
½ teaspoon salt
½ teaspoon freshly ground pepper
1 package (10 ounces) fresh spinach, trimmed and coarsely chopped
¼ cup crumbled feta cheese

1. Cook the pasta according to the package directions.

2. Heat 2 tablespoons of the oil in a large nonstick skillet over high heat. Add the chickpeas and garlic. Cook 3 minutes until the garlic begins to lightly brown, stirring frequently.

3. Reduce the heat and stir in the broth, oregano, salt, and pepper; top with the spinach. Cover and cook 5 minutes until the spinach is wilted.

4. Combine the drained pasta and chickpea mixture in a serving bowl. Toss with the remaining 1 tablespoon oil and sprinkle with the cheese.

SERVES 4

Kilocalories 697 Kc • Protein 24 Gm • Fat 18 Gm • Percent of calories from fat 23% • Cholesterol 15 mg • Dietary Fiber 7 Gm • Sodium 961 mg • Calcium 222 mg

# Spinach and Ravioli Gratin

*A low-fat béchamel (white sauce) tops this dish.*

1½ pounds fresh spinach,
   trimmed
2 cups skim milk
1 small onion, peeled and
   studded with 10 whole cloves
¼ cup all-purpose flour
1 tablespoon unsalted butter

¼ cup snipped fresh chives
¼ teaspoon salt
1 pound mini cheese
   ravioli
1 tablespoon grated Romano
   cheese

1. Place the spinach in a collapsible steamer basket set over simmering water in a wide saucepan. Cover and steam 15 minutes until wilted. Carefully remove the rack from the pot and place in the sink to drain. Cool 10 minutes, then coarsely chop. Place the spinach in the bottom of a 12 × 7½-inch baking dish. Set aside.

2. Combine the milk and onion in a medium saucepan. Bring to a boil over medium heat, and cook 1 minute, stirring constantly. Remove from the heat and let cool. Strain through a sieve into a 2-cup measure; discard the onion.

3. Place the flour in the same medium saucepan. Gradually add the milk, stirring with a whisk until blended. Bring to a boil. Reduce the heat, and simmer 2 minutes or until thickened, stirring constantly. Add the butter and cook 1 minute until it melts, stirring constantly. Remove from the heat and add the chives and salt.

4. Preheat the oven to 400°.

5. Cook the ravioli according to package directions. Drain and spoon onto the spinach. Pour the sauce over the mixture and sprinkle with the cheese. Bake, uncovered, 20 to 25 minutes or until lightly browned.

SERVES 4

Kilocalories 520 Kc • Protein 28 Gm • Fat 20 Gm • Percent of calories from fat 33%
• Cholesterol 52 mg • Dietary Fiber 8 Gm • Sodium 822 mg • Calcium 614 mg

# Spaghettini Asian Style

3 tablespoons dark sesame oil
2 garlic cloves, minced
1½ tablespoons minced fresh
   ginger
16 frozen cooked jumbo
   shrimp, thawed and cut in half

6 cups (packed) shredded
   Chinese or napa cabbage
¾ teaspoon salt
1 pound spaghettini pasta

1. Heat 2 tablespoons of the oil in a large nonstick skillet over low heat. Add the garlic and ginger and cook 1 minute. Add the shrimp and cook 1 minute longer, stirring constantly. Remove the shrimp with a slotted spoon; cover loosely with foil, and set aside.

2. Add the cabbage and salt to the skillet. Cover and cook 5 minutes, stirring once.

3. Cook the pasta according to the package directions. Place the pasta in a serving bowl. Top with the cabbage and shrimp and drizzle with the remaining 1 tablespoon oil. Serve immediately.

SERVES 4

Kilocalories 589 Kc • Protein 28 Gm • Fat 12 Gm • Percent of calories from fat 18% • Cholesterol 0 mg • Dietary Fiber 6 Gm • Sodium 879 mg • Calcium 102 mg

# Swiss Chard-Stuffed Shells

*Fresh tomato sauce is great in season, but during the winter months 3 cups of your favorite tomato sauce may be substituted.*

**24 jumbo pasta shells**

*Filling:*

**2 cups (packed) Swiss chard leaves**
**½ medium onion, cut in half**
**1 tablespoon olive oil**
**1 can (15 ounces) chickpeas, drained and rinsed**
**½ cup part-skim ricotta cheese**
**¼ cup grated Romano cheese**
**1 large egg**
**½ teaspoon salt**

**¼ teaspoon freshly ground pepper**

*Sauce:*

**1 tablespoon olive oil**
**3 tablespoons chopped onion**
**1½ pounds ripe tomatoes, chopped (3½ cups)**
**½ teaspoon salt**
**3 tablespoons chopped fresh flat-leaf parsley**
**2 ounces thinly sliced part-skim mozzarella**

1. Cook the pasta according to the package directions. Drain and set aside.

2. To prepare the filling, place the chard and onion in a food processor. Mince by pulsing the motor on and off.

3. Heat the oil in a medium skillet over medium heat. Cook the chard and onions 1 minute until soft. Cool.

4. Add the chard mixture to the food processor with the remaining filling ingredients. Process 20 seconds until the mixture is smooth.

5. To prepare the sauce, heat the oil in the same skillet over medium heat. Add the onion and cook 1 minute until soft. Add the tomatoes and salt. Cook 8 minutes, stirring frequently. Stir in the parsley.

6. Preheat the oven to 350°. Pour 1 cup of the sauce into a 12 × 7½ - inch baking dish. Spoon a heaping tablespoon of the filling into each shell and arrange in the dish in a single layer. Spoon the remaining sauce over the shells. Top with the mozzarella. Cover and bake for 20 minutes. Uncover and bake 10 minutes longer. Serve immediately.

SERVES 6

**Variation:** Add ⅛ teaspoon grated nutmeg to the filling ingredients. Spoon the filling into a thawed 9-inch frozen pie shell. Sprinkle with 2 tablespoons grated Parmesan cheese. Bake in a 375° oven about 40 minutes until lightly browned.

Kilocalories 331 Kc • Protein 16 Gm • Fat 11 Gm • Percent of calories from fat 29% • Cholesterol 49 mg • Dietary Fiber 7 Gm • Sodium 924 mg • Calcium 192 mg

# Baked Macaroni with Kale

*Any frozen chopped leafy green may be substituted.*

8 ounces elbow macaroni
2 cups diced carrots
1 package (10 ounces) frozen chopped kale
1½ cups shredded low-fat Cheddar cheese (about 6 ounces)

1 tablespoon unsalted butter
½ teaspoon salt
¼ teaspoon freshly ground pepper
1 cup evaporated skimmed milk
1 tablespoon all-purpose flour

1. Bring a large pot of salted water to a boil. Add the macaroni and vegetables and cook 8 minutes until the macaroni is al dente; drain.

2. Preheat the oven to 450°.

3. Return the mixture to the same pot and combine with the cheese, butter, salt, and pepper.

4. Whisk ¼ cup of the milk with the flour in a small bowl. Stir into the macaroni mixture. Add the remaining ¾ cup milk.

5. Spoon the mixture into an 11 × 7-inch baking dish coated with cooking spray. Bake 18 to 20 minutes until lightly brown and bubbly.

SERVES 4

Kilocalories 536 Kc • Protein 32 Gm • Fat 9 Gm • Percent of calories from fat 15% • Cholesterol 24 mg • Dietary Fiber 9 Gm • Sodium 664 mg • Calcium 787 mg

# Bucatini with Chinese Long Beans and Bok Choy

*Chinese long beans look like super-long, thin green beans and are available in Asian markets.*

2 cups Chinese long beans (about 8 ounces)
1 pound bucatini pasta
2 cups chopped bok choy

3 tablespoons dark sesame oil
3 large garlic cloves, minced
½ teaspoon red pepper flakes
½ teaspoon salt

1. Bring a large pot of salted water to a boil. Cook the long beans for 7 minutes. Remove with a slotted spoon and place in a large serving bowl; cover with foil.

2. Add the pasta to the boiling water and cook according to the package directions, adding the bok choy during the last 2 minutes of cooking. Drain and place in the bowl with the beans.

3. Heat the oil over medium heat in a medium nonstick skillet. Cook the garlic and red pepper flakes 1 minute; stir in the salt. Pour the garlic mixture over the pasta mixture in the bowl, tossing to coat.

SERVES 4

Kilocalories 621 Kc • Protein 23 Gm • Fat 13 Gm • Percent of calories from fat 18% • Cholesterol 0 mg • Dietary Fiber 3 Gm • Sodium 311 mg • Calcium 96 mg

# Rigatoni with Arugula, Red Onion, and Pine Nuts

1 pound rigatoni pasta
3 tablespoons extra-virgin olive oil
2 cups thinly sliced red onion
4 cups (packed) arugula, coarsely chopped

1 tablespoon balsamic vinegar
½ teaspoon salt
¼ teaspoon freshly ground pepper
2 tablespoons toasted pignoli nuts

1. Cook the pasta according to the package directions, reserving ½ cup of the pasta water.

2. Meanwhile, heat 2 tablespoons of the oil in a large nonstick skillet over medium-high heat. Add the onion and cook 5 minutes, stirring frequently. Add the arugula, vinegar, salt, and pepper, stirring to combine. Cook 1 to 2 minutes until the arugula is wilted.

3. Combine the pasta and the remaining 1 tablespoon oil in a large serving bowl; add the arugula mixture and toss, adding the reserved pasta water if necessary. Sprinkle with the pine nuts. Serve immediately.

SERVES 4

Kilocalories 570 Kc • Protein 17 Gm • Fat 15 Gm • Percent of calories from fat 23%
• Cholesterol 0 mg • Dietary Fiber 4 Gm • Sodium 307 mg • Calcium 70 mg

# Farfalle with Salmon and Radicchio

1 pound farfalle pasta
2 tablespoons unsalted butter
1 tablespoon olive oil
½ cup minced shallots
1 cup shredded radicchio lettuce
1 cup snow peas (about 3
    ounces), halved diagonally

½ cup chicken broth
½ teaspoon freshly ground
    pepper
½ cup 1% milk
1 tablespoon all-purpose flour
8 ounces sliced smoked salmon,
    cut into 1-inch strips

1. Cook the pasta according to the package directions.

2. Combine the butter and oil in a large nonstick skillet. Cook over medium-high heat until the butter melts.

3. Add the shallots and cook 3 minutes. Stir in the radicchio and snow peas and cook 3 minutes longer, stirring frequently.

4. Stir in the broth and pepper. Cook 3 minutes. Whisk the milk and flour together in a small bowl until smooth. Add to the radicchio mixture in the skillet; cook over medium heat, stirring constantly until thickened and bubbly. Pour the sauce over the pasta. Add the salmon, toss, and serve.

SERVES 4

Kilocalories 609 Kc • Protein 27 Gm • Fat 14 Gm • Percent of calories from fat 22%
• Cholesterol 31 mg • Dietary Fiber 4 Gm • Sodium 485 mg • Calcium 81 mg

# Linguine Primavera with Arugula

1 tablespoon olive oil
2 cups (4 ounces) cremini
   mushrooms, sliced
1 yellow squash, cut into julienne
   strips (about 1 cup)
2 large garlic cloves, minced
½ teaspoon red pepper flakes
2 cups cherry tomatoes, cut in
   half (or 2 cups coarsely
   chopped plum tomatoes)
2 cups (packed) arugula, chopped
½ cup frozen tiny peas
½ teaspoon salt
1½ cups chicken broth
1 cup evaporated skimmed
   milk
4 ounces green beans, trimmed
   and cut into 1-inch pieces
   (1 cup)
½ cup diced carrots
1 pound linguine pasta
¼ cup grated Parmesan
   cheese

1. Heat the oil in a large nonstick skillet over medium heat. Add the mushrooms and cook 3 minutes, stirring occasionally, until softened. Add the squash, garlic, and pepper and cook 2 minutes longer. Add the tomatoes, arugula, peas, and salt, cover, and cook 5 minutes, stirring occasionally. Place the mixture in a large serving bowl and cover with foil.

2. Bring the broth and milk to a boil in a saucepan over medium heat. Add the green beans and carrots; reduce the heat, cover and cook 5 minutes until tender. Drain and add to the vegetables in the serving bowl.

3. Cook the pasta according to the package directions. Drain and toss with the vegetables in the bowl. Sprinkle with the cheese and serve immediately.

SERVES 6

Kilocalories 412 Kc • Protein 18 Gm • Fat 6 Gm • Percent of calories from fat 13%
• Cholesterol 7 mg • Dietary Fiber 5 Gm • Sodium 353 mg • Calcium 217 mg

# Long Fusilli with Cabbage, Onions, and Peas

*Although I prefer savoy cabbage for this dish, green, red or napa cabbage may be used.*

2 cups shredded savoy cabbage
2 cups thinly sliced red onion
3 tablespoons olive oil
1 package (10 ounces) frozen tiny
   peas, thawed

1 pound long fusilli pasta
½ cup grated Parmesan cheese
½ teaspoon freshly ground
   pepper
¼ teaspoon salt

1. Combine the cabbage, onion, and 2 tablespoons of the oil in a large nonstick skillet. Cover and cook over low heat 10 minutes. Uncover and increase the heat to medium. Cook 3 minutes, stirring frequently. Stir in the peas and cook 2 minutes longer. Cover and keep warm.

2. Cook the pasta according to the package directions. Drain the pasta, reserving ¼ cup water, and place the pasta in a serving bowl. Toss with the remaining 1 tablespoon oil, cheese, pepper, salt, and then the cabbage mixture. Add the reserved water, if necessary, and serve immediately.

SERVES 4

Kilocalories 240 Kc • Protein 10 Gm • Fat 14 Gm • Percent of calories from fat 52%
• Cholesterol 13 mg • Dietary Fiber 6 Gm • Sodium 389 mg • Calcium 172 mg

# Linguine with White Clam Sauce and Chicory

*This is a very easy dish to make, providing your fishmonger shucks the clams.*

1 pound linguine pasta
3 tablespoons olive oil
5 large garlic cloves, minced
2 cups (packed) chopped
   chicory

1 cup chopped fresh flat-leaf
   parsley
½ teaspoon salt
3 dozen littleneck clams, shucked
   (reserve liquor)

1. Cook the pasta according to the package directions.

2. Heat the oil in a medium skillet over medium heat. Add the garlic and cook 30 seconds. Add the chicory, cover, and cook 3 minutes. Stir in the parsley, salt, clams, and liquor and cook 4 minutes until the clams are opaque.

3. Place the drained pasta in a large serving bowl. Add the clam mixture, toss, and serve.

SERVES 4

Kilocalories 631 Kc • Protein 29 Gm • Fat 14 Gm • Percent of calories from fat 19%
• Cholesterol 27 mg • Dietary Fiber 12 Gm • Sodium 454 mg • Calcium 310 mg

# Chinese Cabbage Wontons in Soy Sauce

*Oat bran lends not only fiber but a wonderfully nutty flavor to these wontons.*

3 tablespoons dark sesame oil
1 cup finely chopped Chinese or napa cabbage
½ cup mashed drained silken tofu
¼ cup oat bran
¼ cup plain dried bread crumbs
½ cup rolled oats
1½ teaspoons chili paste with garlic
40 wonton wrappers

1 can (15 ounces) straw mushrooms, drained
¼ cup reduced-sodium soy sauce
2 tablespoons dark brown sugar
1 tablespoon toasted sesame seeds
2 teaspoons minced peeled fresh ginger
3 scallions, thinly sliced, for garnish

1. Heat 1 tablespoon of the oil in a small nonstick skillet over medium heat. Add the cabbage and cook 3 minutes, stirring frequently.

2. Combine the tofu, oat bran, bread crumbs, oats, and chili paste in a medium bowl. Stir in the cabbage.

3. Place 1 rounded tablespoon of the cabbage mixture in the center of each of 20 wonton wrappers. Dip a pastry brush in water and moisten the edges of each wrapper.

4. Place 1 of the remaining wonton wrappers over each filling and press the edges together with a fork. Cover the stuffed wontons with damp paper towels.

5. To make the sauce, combine the mushrooms, soy, brown sugar, seeds, and ginger in a small saucepan with ½ cup of water; bring to a boil. Remove from the heat, cover, and keep warm.

6. Cook the wontons 4 minutes in a large pot of boiling water. Remove with a slotted spoon to a serving plate. Spoon the sauce over the wontons. Garnish with the scallions and serve immediately.

SERVES 4

Kilocalories 649 Kc • Protein 22 Gm • Fat 18 Gm • Percent of calories from fat 24% • Cholesterol 7 mg • Dietary Fiber 6 Gm • Sodium 1598 mg • Calcium 186 mg

# Thin Linguine with Mussels

*As a child I called thin linguine* linguine fini. *Some pasta brands today use the term* linguine piccole, *which means "small linguine."*

1 pound thin linguine pasta
2 tablespoons olive oil
2 cups finely chopped beet
  greens
4 large garlic cloves, minced
½ teaspoon dried oregano

¼ teaspoon red pepper flakes
¼ teaspoon salt
2 pounds mussels, washed,
  scrubbed, and bearded
  (discard open mussels)
½ cup dry white wine

1. Cook the pasta according to the package directions.

2. Heat the oil in a large nonstick skillet over medium heat. Add the greens, garlic, oregano, red pepper flakes, and salt and cook 2 minutes, stirring frequently.

3. Add the mussels and wine, cover, and cook 5 minutes, shaking the pan occasionally. (Discard the mussels that haven't opened.) Remove the pan from the heat.

4. Place the pasta in a large serving bowl; top with the mussel mixture and juices. Serve immediately.

SERVES 4

Kilocalories 711 Kc • Protein 43 Gm • Fat 14 Gm • Percent of calories from fat 18%
• Cholesterol 64 mg • Dietary Fiber 4 Gm • Sodium 909 mg • Calcium 141 mg

# Lasagne with Spinach and Feta Cheese

1½ cups part-skim ricotta
    cheese
1¼ cups crumbled feta cheese
    (about 6 ounces)
8 ounces silken tofu, drained
3 packages (10 ounces each)
    frozen chopped spinach,
    thawed but not drained
1 cup thinly sliced scallions

3 tablespoons chopped kalamata
    olives
2 tablespoons snipped fresh dill
¼ teaspoon salt
¼ teaspoon freshly ground
    pepper
¼ teaspoon grated nutmeg
9 curly lasagna noodles
2 cups thinly sliced tomatoes

1. Puree the ricotta, feta, and tofu in a food processor. Place in a large bowl and combine with the spinach, scallions, olives, dill, salt, pepper, and nutmeg.

2. Preheat the oven to 350°.

3. Cook the pasta according to the package directions. Drain well. Alternately layer the noodles and the cheese mixture in a 13 × 9-inch baking dish, coated with vegetable oil spray, ending with the cheese mixture. Top with the tomato slices. Bake 30 minutes. Let the lasagne stand 10 minutes before serving.

SERVES 6

Kilocalories 380 Kc • Protein 24 Gm • Fat 16 Gm • Percent of calories from fat 36% • Cholesterol 55 mg • Dietary Fiber 6 Gm • Sodium 908 mg • Calcium 579 mg

# Perciatelli with Mizuna and Roasted Peppers

*Mizuna reminds me of ruchetta, a spikey-leafed, tiny bitter green more pungent than arugula. To date, I've only found ruchetta in Italy.*

6 yellow bell peppers
¼ cup chiffonade of basil
1 tablespoon extra-virgin
   olive oil
½ teaspoon salt

¼ teaspoon freshly ground
   pepper
1 pound perciatelli pasta
2 cups (packed) coarsely
   chopped mizuna

1. Preheat the oven to 500°. Place the peppers in a 9-inch square baking pan (if they don't fit, use an 11 × 7-inch pan). Roast for 10 to 15 minutes, turning once, until the skins are blackened and blistered. Remove from the oven and cover with foil. Let them stand 20 minutes. Reserve the juice in the pan.

2. Pierce the peppers to let the steam and water escape. Peel, seed, and cut the peppers into ¼-inch strips. Place in a large serving bowl with the basil, oil, salt, pepper, and the reserved pepper juice.

3. Cook the pasta according to the package directions. Drain and combine with the mizuna. Stir in the pepper mixture, toss, and serve.

SERVES 4

Kilocalories 483 Kc • Protein 16 Gm • Fat 5 Gm • Percent of calories from fat 10%
• Cholesterol 0 mg • Dietary Fiber 5 Gm • Sodium 304 mg • Calcium 51 mg

# Ziti with Grilled Chicken and Watercress

*Lots of southwestern flavor.*

2 tablespoons chili powder
1 teaspoon garlic powder
8 ounces boneless, skinless
 chicken breast tenderloins
1 cup diced tomatoes
2 cups (packed) chopped
 watercress

¼ cup chopped fresh cilantro
2 tablespoons olive oil
½ teaspoon salt
1 pound ziti pasta

1. Combine the chili powder and garlic powder in a small sealable plastic bag. Add a few pieces of chicken at a time and shake to coat.

2. Heat the stovetop or oven grill, coated with vegetable oil spray, over medium heat. Cook the chicken 3 minutes on each side. Remove and cut into 1-inch pieces.

3. Combine the tomatoes, watercress, cilantro, oil, and salt in a large serving bowl.

4. Cook the pasta according to the package directions. Drain and place in the bowl. Toss gently with the tomato mixture. Top with the chicken and toss again before serving.

SERVES 4

Kilocalories 629 Kc • Protein 29 Gm • Fat 16 Gm • Percent of calories from fat 23%
• Cholesterol 28 mg • Dietary Fiber 4 Gm • Sodium 350 mg • Calcium 62 mg

# Rotelli with Raw Tomato Sauce and Mustard Greens

*Ricotta salata is a salty Italian sheep's milk cheese. It's denser and more flavorful than ricotta cheese and adds a special touch to this summer dish.*

3 cups diced tomatoes
¼ cup chopped fresh basil
¼ cup chopped onion
2 tablespoons extra-virgin olive oil
1 tablespoon balsamic vinegar
¾ teaspoon salt

¼ teaspoon freshly ground pepper
1 package (10 ounces) frozen mustard greens
1 pound rotelli pasta
¼ cup shredded ricotta salata cheese or coarsely grated Romano cheese

1. Combine the tomatoes, basil, onion, oil, vinegar, salt, and pepper in a bowl. Let the mixture stand, covered, 2 hours. (This can be made ahead and refrigerated. Bring to room temperature before serving.)

2. Bring salted water to a boil for the pasta. Add the frozen mustard greens and cook about 7 minutes, separating the block with a long-handled fork. Add the pasta and cook according to the package directions. Drain and place the mixture in a serving bowl. Add the tomato mixture and toss. Sprinkle with the cheese.

SERVES 4

Kilocalories 559 Kc • Protein 20 Gm • Fat 11 Gm • Percent of calories from fat 18%
• Cholesterol 6 mg • Dietary Fiber 6 Gm • Sodium 562 mg • Calcium 169 mg

# Orecchiette with Broccoli Raab

2 tablespoons olive oil
4 large garlic cloves, minced
¾ teaspoon red pepper flakes
1 teaspoon salt
1 pound orecchiette pasta
1 bunch (about 1¼ pounds)

broccoli raab, trimmed and
  roughly chopped
8 kalamata olives, pitted and
  sliced
Grated Romano cheese, optional

1. Heat the oil in a small nonstick skillet over medium heat. Add the garlic and red pepper flakes and cook 30 seconds or until the garlic begins to brown. Remove from the heat and stir in the salt.

2. Cook the pasta according to the package directions, reserving ½ cup cooking water. Add the broccoli raab during the last 5 minutes of cooking time. Drain and place the mixture in a large serving bowl. Add the oil mixture and olives; toss to coat. Add the reserved pasta water, if necessary for a moister dish. Sprinkle with the cheese, if desired.

SERVES 4

Kilocalories 523 Kc • Protein 16 Gm • Fat 10 Gm • Percent of calories from fat 17% • Cholesterol 0 mg • Dietary Fiber 7 Gm • Sodium 708 mg • Calcium 228 mg

# Ravioli with Tomato Mushroom Sauce and Fresh Arugula

1 tablespoon olive oil
6 ounces (3½ cups) sliced cremini
   mushrooms
1 large garlic clove, minced
1 can (28 ounces) Italian-style
   tomatoes and juice, pureed
½ teaspoon salt

1 tablespoon fresh marjoram
   (1 teaspoon dried)
1 box (18) large cheese ravioli
2 cups (packed) slivered arugula
¼ cup grated Parmesan
   cheese

1. Heat the oil in a large nonstick skillet over medium heat. Add the mushrooms and cook 2 minutes, stirring frequently; add the garlic and cook 1 minute longer. Reduce the heat and add the tomatoes and salt. Simmer 20 minutes, stirring occasionally. Add the marjoram and remove from the heat.

2. Cook the ravioli according to the package directions. Place in a serving bowl and toss them with the sauce. Top with the arugula and sprinkle with the cheese. Serve immediately.

SERVES 6

Kilocalories 224 Kc • Protein 10 Gm • Fat 10 Gm • Percent of calories from fat 39%
• Cholesterol 20 mg • Dietary Fiber 3 Gm • Sodium 712 mg • Calcium 185 mg

# Penne with Roasted Beets and Beet Greens

*Penne rigate is a ridged pen-shaped pasta. It's a little chewier than the smooth penne, adding more texture to the dish.*

1 bunch beets with greens
1 pound penne rigate pasta
3 tablespoons olive oil
¼ cup chiffonade of fresh basil
¼ teaspoon salt

⅛ teaspoon freshly ground
  pepper
1 cup shredded Parmesan
  cheese

1. Preheat the oven to 400°.

2. Separate the beet greens from the beets; rinse, drain, and chop them. Set aside.

3. Rinse the beet roots; trim the tops and bottoms. Place on aluminum foil and wrap tightly. Bake 1 to 1½ hours until they are tender when pierced with a skewer.

4. When the beets are cool enough to handle, peel and cut into julienne strips; set aside.

5. Cook the pasta according to the package directions, adding the beet greens during the last 5 minutes of cooking. Drain the pasta mixture and place in a large serving bowl; toss with the oil. Add the beets, basil, salt, and pepper and toss again. Top with the Parmesan and serve.

SERVES 4

Kilocalories 703 Kc • Protein 28 Gm • Fat 19 Gm • Percent of calories from fat 25%
• Cholesterol 25 mg • Dietary Fiber 10 Gm • Sodium 846 mg • Calcium 419 mg

# Gnocchi with Chickpeas, Collards, and Cheddar

*Chickpeas, legumes, add protein power to this dish.*

1 pound gnocchi (dried pasta)
3 tablespoons oil
1 can (15 ounces) chickpeas, drained
3 large garlic cloves, minced
½ cup chicken broth
½ teaspoon dried oregano
½ teaspoon salt
½ teaspoon freshly ground pepper
8 cups (packed) chopped fresh collard greens
¼ cup shredded Cheddar cheese

1. Cook the pasta according to the package directions.

2. Heat 2 tablespoons of the oil in a large nonstick skillet over high heat. Add the chickpeas and garlic. Cook 3 minutes until the garlic begins to lightly brown, stirring frequently.

3. Reduce the heat and stir in the broth, oregano, salt, and pepper; add the collards. Cover and cook 5 minutes until the collards are wilted.

4. Combine the drained pasta and chickpea mixture in a large serving bowl. Toss with the remaining 1 tablespoon oil and sprinkle with the cheese.

SERVES 4

Kilocalories 477 Kc • Protein 15 Gm • Fat 17 Gm • Percent of calories from fat 30%
• Cholesterol 16 mg • Dietary Fiber 8 Gm • Sodium 798 mg • Calcium 129 mg

# Radiatore with Zucchini, Escarole, and Mint

1 cup chicken broth
4 medium zucchini, sliced (about 4 cups)
3 tablespoons olive oil
3 cups finely chopped escarole
½ cup chopped fresh mint
¼ teaspoon salt

¼ teaspoon freshly ground pepper
1 pound radiatore pasta
Grated Parmesan cheese, optional
Fresh mint sprigs for garnish

1. Combine the broth and zucchini in a large skillet over medium heat. Cover and cook 10 minutes. Uncover and cook 10 minutes longer, stirring frequently. Stir in 2 tablespoons of the oil, the escarole, mint, salt, and pepper. Cook 3 minutes, cover, and set aside.

2. Cook the pasta according to the package directions. Place the pasta in a large serving bowl and toss with the remaining 1 tablespoon oil. Add the zucchini mixture and toss again. Sprinkle with cheese, if desired, and garnish with mint.

SERVES 4

Kilocalories 555 Kc • Protein 17 Gm • Fat 13 Gm • Percent of calories from fat 21% • Cholesterol 1 mg • Dietary Fiber 6 Gm • Sodium 190 mg • Calcium 69 mg

# Conchiglie with Spinach Pesto and Potatoes

*Pasta "shells" come in three sizes; small, medium, and large. Small shells are great for soups, large for stuffing, but medium are best suited for chunky pasta sauces.*

2 cups (packed) chopped fresh
    spinach
⅓ cup chicken broth
⅓ cup grated Romano cheese
¼ cup 1% milk
3 tablespoons olive oil
1 tablespoon pignoli nuts
2 garlic cloves

1 teaspoon salt
½ teaspoon freshly ground black
    pepper
1½ pounds potatoes, peeled and
    cut into 1-inch cubes (about 4
    cups)
1 pound medium conchiglie (shell
    pasta)

1. To prepare the pesto, combine all of the ingredients except the potatoes and shells in a food processor. Process 30 seconds until creamy. Set aside.

2. Bring a large pot of salted water to a boil. Add the potatoes and cook 2 minutes. Stir in the pasta and cook according to the package directions.

3. Drain the pasta mixture and toss in a large serving bowl with the pesto. Serve immediately.

SERVES 4

**Variation:** Arugula Pesto: Substitute arugula for the spinach, 2 tablespoons walnuts instead of the pignoli, and add ¼ cup chopped fresh flat-leaf parsley.

Kilocalories 711 Kc • Protein 23 Gm • Fat 16 Gm • Percent of calories from fat 20% • Cholesterol 9 mg • Dietary Fiber 6 Gm • Sodium 749 mg • Calcium 166 mg

# Spinach Fettuccine (Tagliatelle) with Cherry Tomato Sauce

*You will need a manual pasta machine with a fettuccine cutter for this recipe. After you make the pasta, you'll probably be too tired to make a sauce, so I'm including a recipe for one of the quickest and easiest to make, other than a raw tomato sauce. Of course, you can use your own homemade sauce. You'll need about 2 cups for this amount of pasta.*

*Pasta:*

8 ounces fresh spinach, stems
    removed
2½ cups unbleached all-purpose
    flour
3 large eggs, lightly beaten
¼ teaspoon salt

Grated Parmesan cheese,
    optional

*Sauce:*

1 teaspoon olive oil
1 large garlic clove, minced
2 pints cherry tomatoes, rinsed,
    dried, and halved
1 teaspoon fresh marjoram (or
    herb of choice)
½ teaspoon salt
½ teaspoon freshly ground
    pepper

1. To prepare the pasta, add the spinach to salted boiling water and cook 3 minutes. Drain and cool; squeeze out the excess water, then place in a clean kitchen towel and squeeze again. Puree the spinach in a food processor. Add the flour, eggs, and salt to the food processor and pulse to combine. Process until a ball forms, adding a little water, if necessary. Process an additional 30 seconds to knead. Place the dough in a bowl, cover, and let it rest 30 minutes.

2. To prepare the sauce, heat the oil in a large nonstick skillet over medium heat. Add the garlic and cook about 30 seconds until lightly browned. Add the tomatoes, marjoram, salt, and pepper and cook 10 minutes, stirring occasionally.

3. Cut the dough into eighths and cover. Flatten one piece of dough into a rectangle. Roll the dough through a manual pasta machine on the first setting. Lightly dust with flour and fold the dough into thirds and put through the machine again. Do this 3 or 4 more times until the dough is

smooth (this also continues the kneading process). Then run the dough through the machine once on each notch up to and including number 6. Let the sheets dry on the counter 20 to 30 minutes (this prevents it from sticking when you are cutting the dough).

4. Attach the fettuccine cutter to the machine. Pass each sheet of pasta through the cutter. If the sheets are still a little sticky, dust lightly with flour. Place the pasta strands on lengths of paper towels, separating the strands if necessary. The pasta may remain on the counter up to 1 hour before cooking.

5. Cook the pasta in a large pot of boiling salted water for 2 to 3 minutes, until tender. Drain and serve immediately with the sauce and grated cheese, if desired.

SERVES 4

**Variation:** Frozen Chopped Spinach Pasta: Use ½ package (10 ounces) frozen chopped spinach in place of the fresh; cook and follow the same instructions to prepare the pasta, adding ⅛ teaspoon of grated nutmeg to the ingredients in the food processor. If necessary, add cold water, 1 tablespoon at a time, through the feed tube until a ball forms. Using frozen spinach doesn't alter the flavor of this recipe.

Kilocalories 411 Kc • Protein 16 Gm • Fat 7 Gm • Percent of calories from fat 14% • Cholesterol 159 mg • Dietary Fiber 7 Gm • Sodium 550 mg • Calcium 179 mg

# Whole Wheat Pasta Fagioli with Escarole

*My Mom's pasta fagioli is the best. This variation combines pasta with cannellini beans, but occasionally she used chickpeas in this tasty vegetarian dish.*

1 tablespoon olive oil
2 garlic cloves, minced
1½ cups chopped, drained
   canned tomatoes
½ teaspoon salt
½ teaspoon dried
   oregano

8 ounces whole wheat penne
   pasta
2 cups finely chopped escarole
1 can (15 ounces) cannellini
   beans, rinsed and drained
¼ cup grated Romano cheese

1. Heat the oil in a 3-quart saucepan over medium heat. Add the garlic and cook 30 seconds until softened. Add the tomatoes, salt, and oregano and cook 5 minutes, stirring occasionally.

2. Add 3½ cups water; cover and bring to a boil. Stir in the pasta and cook according to the package directions. During the last 5 minutes of cooking, stir in the escarole. Add the beans and cook until heated through. Place in serving bowls and sprinkle with the cheese.

SERVES 4

**Kilocalories 412 Kc • Protein 20 Gm • Fat 6 Gm • Percent of calories from fat 14% • Cholesterol 6 mg • Dietary Fiber 8 Gm • Sodium 1087 mg • Calcium 184 mg**

# Tortellini with Cabbage and Capers

4 cups shredded cabbage
1 cup thinly sliced onion
1 cup chicken broth
3 tablespoons olive oil

1 tablespoon rinsed capers
½ teaspoon salt
¼ teaspoon pepper
1 pound cheese tortellini

1. Combine the cabbage, onion, and broth in a large nonstick skillet. Cover and cook 10 minutes over medium heat, stirring occasionally. Uncover, add the oil, capers, salt, and pepper, and cook 3 to 5 minutes longer, stirring frequently, until the cabbage and onions are lightly browned.

2. Cook the tortellini according to the package directions. Drain and place in a serving bowl. Toss with the cabbage mixture and serve immediately.

SERVES 4

Kilocalories 480 Kc • Protein 20 Gm • Fat 19 Gm • Percent of calories from fat 35% • Cholesterol 61 mg • Dietary Fiber 6 Gm • Sodium 848 mg • Calcium 242 mg

# Vegetable Lasagne Rolls

*This is a delicious vegetarian entree, but these rich lasagna bundles are also terrific as a side dish.*

*Tomato Sauce:*

1 can (16 ounces) Italian-style
    tomatoes, chopped, with juice
1 tablespoon minced fresh basil
1 teaspoon sugar
¼ teaspoon salt
¼ teaspoon freshly ground pepper

*Filling:*

2 tablespoons olive oil
½ cup minced onion
½ cup minced carrot
1 cup finely chopped green bell
    pepper

2 garlic cloves, finely minced
1 cup finely chopped yellow
    squash
1 cup finely chopped zucchini
3 cups shredded and chopped
    radicchio
½ teaspoon salt
½ teaspoon freshly ground pepper
1 cup shredded domestic Havarti
    cheese (about 4 ounces)
8 lasagna noodles, cooked
2 tablespoons grated Parmesan
    cheese

1. Combine all of the sauce ingredients in a medium saucepan. Simmer over low heat for 30 minutes, stirring occasionally.

2. Preheat the oven to 350°.

3. To prepare the filling, heat the oil in a large nonstick skillet over medium heat. Cook the onion, carrot, green pepper, garlic, squash, and zucchini 5 to 7 minutes, until tender. Stir in the radicchio, cover, and cook 2 minutes longer, until wilted. Remove the pan from the heat. Stir in the salt and pepper; cook for 10 minutes. Toss with the Havarti cheese.

4. Spread a scant ½ cup vegetable-cheese mixture on each length of lasagna noodle. Roll it up, starting at the short end. Spoon 1 cup of tomato sauce on the bottom of an 11 × 7-inch baking dish. Place each pasta roll, seam side down, in the dish. Spoon another cup of tomato sauce over the top to cover (save the remaining 1 cup of sauce for another use). Sprinkle with Parmesan cheese, cover with foil, and bake 20 minutes. Uncover and bake 10 minutes longer until heated through and bubbly.

SERVES 4 (MAKES 8 ROLLS AND 3 CUPS SAUCE)

Kilocalories 648 Kc • Protein 21 Gm • Fat 30 Gm • Percent of calories from fat 41%
• Cholesterol 46 mg • Dietary Fiber 9 Gm • Sodium 2349 mg • Calcium 407 mg

# Garganelli with Asparagus and Radicchio

*Garganelli are little squares of pasta that have been rolled and sealed on the diagonal. If they are unavailable in your supermarket, you can substitute penne or ziti.*

1 pound asparagus, trimmed and peeled
2 small firm heads radicchio, quartered (about 8 ounces)
2 tablespoons olive oil
½ teaspoon kosher or coarse salt
1 pound garganelli pasta
3 tablespoons vegetable broth
2 tablespoons half-and-half
Freshly ground pepper

1. Preheat the oven to 425°.

2. Place the asparagus and radicchio in a single layer in a 15 × 10-inch jelly roll pan coated with vegetable oil spray. Drizzle with 1 tablespoon of the oil and sprinkle with the salt. Roast 10 minutes. Stir the asparagus and turn the radicchio (with tongs, if you have them); roast 10 minutes longer. Cool slightly. Cut the asparagus on the diagonal into 2-inch pieces and place in a large serving bowl Trim the core from the radicchio, and slice into shreds. Add to the bowl.

3. Cook the pasta according to the package directions and drain.

4. Meanwhile, combine the broth, half-and-half, and pepper in a small saucepan. Bring to a boil over medium-high heat. Reduce the heat to medium and cook until the liquid is reduced by half.

5. Combine the pasta, asparagus, radicchio, broth reduction, and remaining oil in a large serving bowl. Toss and serve immediately.

SERVES 4

Kilocalories 521 Kc • Protein 18 Gm • Fat 10 Gm • Percent of calories from fat 17% • Cholesterol 3 mg • Dietary Fiber 5 Gm • Sodium 321 mg • Calcium 60 mg

# Three-Cheese Vegetable Lasagne

2 teaspoons olive oil
2 cups chopped fresh broccoli
1½ cups thinly sliced carrots
1 cup sliced scallions
½ cup chopped red bell pepper
3 garlic cloves, crushed
½ cup all-purpose flour
3 cups skim milk
½ cup grated Parmesan cheese
¼ teaspoon salt

¼ teaspoon freshly ground
  pepper
1 package (10 ounces) frozen
  chopped collard greens,
  thawed, drained, and squeezed
1½ cups part-skim ricotta cheese
1 cup (4 ounces) shredded part-
  skim mozzarella
12 cooked lasagna noodles

1. Coat a Dutch oven with vegetable oil spray; add the oil, and heat over medium heat. Add the broccoli, carrots, scallions, bell pepper, and garlic. Cook 7 minutes until just tender. Set aside.

2. Place the flour in a medium saucepan. Gradually add the milk, stirring with a wire whisk until blended. Bring to a boil over medium heat, and cook 5 minutes or until thickened, stirring constantly. Add ¼ cup of the Parmesan cheese, the salt, and pepper; cook 1 minute longer, stirring constantly. Remove from the heat and stir in the collards. Reserve 1 cup of the mixture.

3. Preheat the oven to 375°.

4. Combine the ricotta and mozzarella in a medium bowl.

5. Spread ½ cup of the reserved collard mixture in the bottom of a 13 × 9-inch baking pan coated with vegetable oil spray. Arrange 4 noodles over the collard mixture; top with half the cheese mixture, half the vegetable mixture, and half the main collard mixture. Repeat the layers, ending with the remaining 4 noodles. Spread the remaining reserved ½ cup collard mixture over the noodles, and sprinkle with the remaining ¼ cup Parmesan cheese. Cover and bake for 35 minutes. Let the lasagne stand 5 minutes before serving.

SERVES 8

Kilocalories 316 Kc • Protein 20 Gm • Fat 8 Gm • Percent of calories from fat 23% • Cholesterol 24 mg • Dietary Fiber 4 Gm • Sodium 396 mg • Calcium 422 mg

# Pizzocheri

*This is a typical pasta dish from the mountain region (Val d'Aosta) in northern Italy. Buckwheat pasta is available at Italian specialty food stores and health food stores.*

3 medium potatoes (about 1 pound), pared and diced
4 cups finely shredded savoy cabbage
1 pound buckwheat pasta or soba noodles
1 tablespoon oil

2 garlic cloves, sliced
½ cup chicken broth
½ teaspoon salt
4 ounces Taleggio cheese, rind removed and cut into ½-inch cubes (may substitute fontina cheese)

1. Put the potatoes in a large pot of boiling salted water and cook 3 minutes. Add the cabbage and cook 5 minutes longer. Add the noodles and cook according to the package directions.

2. While the pasta is cooking, heat the oil in a small skillet over medium heat. Add the garlic and cook 30 seconds until lightly browned. Remove from the heat and cool slightly. Stir in the broth and salt.

3. Drain the pasta mixture and place in a serving bowl. Toss with the broth mixture and garnish with the cheese cubes. Cover with foil 1 minute until the cheese melts. Toss again and serve immediately.

SERVES 6

Kilocalories 446 Kc • Protein 15 Gm • Fat 11 Gm • Percent of calories from fat 21% • Cholesterol 22 mg • Dietary Fiber 7 Gm • Sodium 412 mg • Calcium 128 mg

# Spinach and Ricotta Gnocchi

*Good friend and cookbook author Michele Scicolone gave me her famous version of this dish. The following is a streamlined facsimile which may turn Michele's hair white. Even this version isn't as low fat as I'd like, but by substituting tomato sauce for the traditional butter topping, you are doing your body a favor.*

2 pounds spinach, trimmed (wet) or 2 packages (10 ounces each) frozen chopped spinach, thawed
1 tablespoon unsalted butter
1 tablespoon olive oil
¼ cup finely chopped onion
1 container (15 ounces) part-skim ricotta cheese
1½ cups plus 2 tablespoons all-purpose flour

1 cup grated Parmesan cheese (4 ounces)
3 large eggs, lightly beaten
¼ teaspoon grated nutmeg
¼ teaspoon salt
¼ teaspoon freshly ground pepper
3 cups homemade tomato sauce
Chopped fresh sage leaves for garnish, optional

1. Place the wet spinach in a large pot. Cover and cook 2 to 3 minutes over medium heat or until wilted and tender. Drain and cool. Place in a clean kitchen towel and squeeze out the excess water. Finely chop the spinach. (If you are using frozen spinach, squeeze out the excess water, but do not cook.)

2. Combine the butter and oil in a medium skillet. Place over medium-low heat 1 to 2 minutes or until the butter melts. Add the onion and cook, stirring occasionally, until softened, about 3 minutes. Stir in the chopped spinach until combined. Remove the mixture from the heat and cool slightly.

3. Combine the ricotta, 1½ cups flour, Parmesan, eggs, nutmeg, salt, and pepper with a wooden spoon in a large bowl. The mixture will be soft.

4. Spread the remaining 2 tablespoons flour on a dinner plate. Lightly flour your hands and shape the gnocchi mixture into balls about ¾ inch in diameter, rolling them lightly in flour if still sticky. Put the gnocchi on

baking sheets lined with wax paper, cover, and refrigerate up to several hours until you are ready to cook them.*

5. Add half the gnocchi to a large pot of boiling salted water, a few at a time to prevent them from sticking. After the gnocchi rise to the surface, cook 1 to 2 minutes longer. Remove the gnocchi with a slotted spoon and place them on a serving platter. Repeat with the remaining gnocchi. Serve with the tomato sauce, heated, and sprinkle with sage, if desired.

SERVES 4

*Gnocchi may be frozen in a single layer. After they are frozen, place half of the gnocchi in each of two large sealable plastic freezer bags. Cook half the gnocchi at a time following the same instructions.

**Kilocalories 703 Kc • Protein 41 Gm • Fat 32 Gm • Percent of calories from fat 40% • Cholesterol 227 mg • Dietary Fiber 12 Gm • Sodium 1521 mg • Calcium 872 mg**

# Fusilli with Mushrooms, Peas, and Arugula

1 tablespoon olive oil
3 slices turkey bacon, finely chopped
½ cup chopped onion
3 cups sliced fresh mushrooms (about 8 ounces)
¼ cup dry vermouth
½ teaspoon salt
¼ teaspoon freshly ground pepper

2 cups vegetable or chicken broth
1 cup fresh or frozen peas
1 tablespoon unsalted butter
1 pound fusilli pasta
⅓ cup grated Parmesan cheese
5 cups chopped arugula,

1. Bring a large pot of water to a boil.

2. Meanwhile, heat the oil in large nonstick skillet over medium heat. Add the bacon and onion and cook 3 to 4 minutes, stirring frequently, until the onion is tender. Stir in the mushrooms, vermouth, salt, and pepper; cover and cook 5 minutes. Uncover and cook 3 minutes longer until the mushrooms are lightly browned.

3. Add the broth, peas, and butter to the skillet; increase the heat to high. Cook about 10 minutes until the liquid is reduced by half.

4. Cook the pasta according to the package directions. Drain and place in a serving bowl. Toss the pasta with the cheese; stir in the arugula and the vegetable mixture and serve immediately.

SERVES 4

Kilocalories 626 Kc • Protein 23 Gm • Fat 13 Gm • Percent of calories from fat 19% • Cholesterol 24 mg • Dietary Fiber 6 Gm • Sodium 605 mg • Calcium 155 mg

# Orzo with Scallops and Spinach

*This is a tasty first course.*

2 tablespoons olive oil
2 tablespoons minced shallots
8 ounces bay scallops
¾ cup clam juice or fish broth

2 tablespoons fresh lemon juice
¼ teaspoon salt
4 cups finely chopped trimmed
 spinach
8 ounces (1¼ cups) orzo

1. Bring a large pot of water to a boil.

2. Meanwhile, heat 1 tablespoon of the oil in a medium skillet over medium heat. Add the shallots and cook for 30 seconds. Add the scallops; cook 1 minute, stirring frequently. Stir in the clam juice, lemon juice, and the salt. Turn the heat to high and bring to a boil. Add the spinach; cover and cook 2 minutes, stirring once.

3. Cook the pasta according to the package directions.

4. Drain the pasta and place in a medium serving bowl. Add the remaining 1 tablespoon of oil and toss. Add the scallop mixture and toss again. Serve immediately.

SERVES 4

Kilocalories 347 Kc • Protein 22 Gm • Fat 9 Gm • Percent of calories from fat 22%
• Cholesterol 30 mg • Dietary Fiber 3 Gm • Sodium 379 mg • Calcium 132 mg

# 6
# Greens and Grains

Grains were cultivated along the Mediterranean and in Palestine and Syria as early as 10,000 B.C. There is evidence at this time of a shift from more primitive nomadic tribes to civilizations based on farming. Villages sprang up and fertility cults worshipping mother-figure goddesses came to be. In Greece, temples were erected in honor of Demeter, the goddess of agriculture and protector of the harvest.

In our contemporary food pyramid, cereals form the base, with the recommendation that they be given a high priority in our diet. Greens are right above them. This chapter explores the combination of these two agrarian treasures—greens and grains. A natural combination, they enrich our diet not only with vitamins and minerals, but also with plenty of fiber.

There are many opportunities to pair greens with common grains like corn, barley, rice, bulgur, and rolled oats. I've also introduced recipes using less familiar grains such as amaranth, millet, quinoa, and oat groats. This chapter includes recipes for main dish meals as well as side dishes.

# Risotto with Radicchio and Smoked Mozzarella (Pressure Cooker/Master Recipe*)

*Risotto is a northern Italian first-course dish usually made with arborio rice. This is a starchy rice, and when it is slowly combined with a liquid, it releases the starch, binds the kernels together, and becomes very creamy. Regular rice may not be substituted, but other varieties of short-grain rice which work well are Vialone Nano, Canaroli, and Japanese sushi rice, which is very inexpensive and may be bought at Asian markets.*

1½ tablespoons olive oil
1 cup thinly sliced leek, white part only
1½ cups arborio rice
3¼ cups vegetable or chicken broth

2 cups shredded radicchio
1 cup shredded smoked mozzarella (about 2½ ounces)
¼ cup grated Parmesan cheese
Salt and freshly ground pepper

1. Heat the oil in an open pressure cooker over medium heat. Add the leeks and cook until soft, about 2 minutes. Stir in the rice to coat.

2. Stir in the broth, the radicchio, and mozzarella. Lock the lid in place and bring to high pressure over high heat. Adjust the heat to maintain the pressure. Cook for 4 minutes. Release the pressure by placing the edge of the pot under running cold water. Remove the lid, tilting it away from you to allow excess steam to escape. Taste the risotto, which should be creamy yet al dente. Stir in the Parmesan cheese. Season with salt and pepper.

SERVES 4

**\*Traditional cooking method (Master Recipe):** Bring the broth to a simmer over low heat. Heat the oil in a dutch oven or wide, heavy saucepan over medium heat. Add the leaks and cook until soft, stirring frequently, about 2 minutes. Stir in the rice to coat. Add ½ cup of the warm broth to rice mixture. Cook, stirring constantly, until the liquid is absorbed. Add another ½ cup of the broth and stir until absorbed. At this point, stir in the radicchio. Add the remaining broth, ½ cup at a time, stirring until the rice is just tender and creamy, 20 to 25 minutes. Remove from the heat and stir in the cheeses, salt, and pepper. Serve immediately.

**Variation 1:** Pumpkin and Kale Risotto: 1 tablespoon olive oil, 1½ cups chopped onion, 1½ cups arborio rice, 3¼ cups chicken broth, 3 cups chopped kale, 1 cup canned pureed pumpkin, 1 teaspoon grated lemon zest, ⅛ teaspoon grated nutmeg, salt and pepper to taste. Follow the master recipe instructions, adding pumpkin and nutmeg, salt, and pepper after the rice has cooked.

**Variation 2:** Cabbage Risotto Milanese: 2 tablespoons unsalted butter, ½ cup chopped onion, ¼ cup chopped shallots, 1½ cups arborio rice, 3¼ cups chicken broth, 4 cups shredded cabbage, ¼ teaspoon saffron powder *or* ½ teaspoon chopped saffron threads, salt and pepper to taste. Cook the onion and shallots in 1 tablespoon of the butter. Follow the master recipe instructions, adding the remaining 1 tablespoon of butter, salt and pepper after the rice is cooked.

**Variation 3:** Spinach and Gruyère Risotto: 1½ tablespoons olive oil, 2 cups chopped onion, 1½ cups arborio rice, 3¼ cups chicken broth, 10 ounces fresh spinach, trimmed and chopped, ½ cup shredded Gruyère or Swiss cheese. Follow the instructions for the master recipe, adding the cheese after the rice is cooked.

**Variation 4:** Risotto Patty Cakes: All of the above recipes can be made into patties and served as a side dish or as a main vegetarian dish on top of steamed or sautéed greens (preferably the same used in the recipe). Cool the risotto and refrigerate 2 hours or until the mixture holds together. Make 3-inch patties or mold with a spoon tightly into ½-cup measures and release onto a baking sheet by inserting a knife around the rim; place the patties or molded rice on a dish or baking sheet; cover and refrigerate up to 24 hours. Coat a large nonstick skillet with vegetable oil spray. Place over medium heat. Add a teaspoon or two of olive oil to the pan and rotate so that the oil lightly covers the bottom of the pan. When the oil is hot, add the patties, pressing down with a spatula. Cook 3 to 4 minutes on each side until browned and crisp. Repeat with the remaining patties.

**Kilocalories 528 Kc • Protein 18 Gm • Fat 10 Gm • Percent of calories from fat 18% • Cholesterol 16 mg • Dietary Fiber 3 Gm • Sodium 309 mg • Calcium 303 mg**

# Baked Wild Mushroom and Mache Risotto

*This is a very easy way to make risotto. It's not quite as creamy as the stovetop or pressure cooker methods, but it's equally delicious.*

1½ tablespoons olive oil
12 ounces wild mushrooms (shiitake, chanterelle, porcini, morel, portobello), chopped
½ cup chopped onion
2 cups chopped mache (arugula or mesclun)

2 cups arborio rice
5 cups chicken or vegetable broth
½ cup grated Parmesan cheese
Salt and freshly ground pepper, optional

1. Preheat the oven to 350°.

2. Heat 1 tablespoon of the oil in a large nonstick skillet over medium heat. Add the mushrooms and onion; cook 8 to 10 minutes, stirring frequently until the mushrooms are browned. Add the mache, cover, and cook 1 to 2 minutes until wilted. Remove the mixture with a slotted spoon to a medium bowl.

3. Add the remaining ½ tablespoon of oil to the skillet; stir in the rice. Cook 2 minutes, stirring constantly. Add 1 cup broth and simmer 3 minutes. Pour the rice into the mushroom mixture, add the cheese and stir to combine. Spoon into an 8- or 9-inch baking dish (2 inches deep). Stir in the remaining 4 cups of broth, taste the mixture, and season with salt and pepper if necessary. Bake about 1 hour or until the liquid is absorbed.

SERVES 4

Kilocalories 626 Kc • Protein 18 Gm • Fat 12 Gm • Percent of calories from fat 18%
• Cholesterol 18 mg • Dietary Fiber 4 Gm • Sodium 292 mg • Calcium 148 mg

# Two-Grain Stuffed Trout

*Oat groats are the whole oat kernel with the husk removed. Steel-cut oats are groats which have been cut into pieces. They are rich in B vitamins and flavor.*

½ cup steel-cut oats
¼ cup bulgur wheat
2 (12-ounce) whole dressed trout
   (boned and heads removed)
2 tablespoons oat flour
½ teaspoon ground red pepper
½ teaspoon ground cumin
½ teaspoon grated nutmeg

½ teaspoon ground ginger
½ cup finely chopped mache or
   watercress
½ cup sliced scallions
1 teaspoon grated fresh ginger
½ teaspoon salt
2 tablespoons olive oil

1. Combine the oats and bulgur wheat with just enough water to cover in a medium saucepan. Bring to a boil over high heat; remove from the heat. Let the saucepan stand, covered, 10 minutes, until the water is absorbed.

2. Preheat the oven to 350°.

3. Rinse the fish and pat it dry with paper towels. Place in a 12 × 7½-inch baking dish coated with vegetable oil spray.

4. Combine the oat flour, pepper, cumin, nutmeg, and ground ginger in a small bowl. Rub the fish, inside and out, with some of the oat flour mixture.

5. Combine the remaining oat flour mixture, mache, scallions, fresh ginger, and salt; spoon equal amounts into the cavities of the fish. Close with kitchen string and drizzle with oil.

6. Bake, uncovered, about 25 minutes, until the fish is opaque.

SERVES 4

Kilocalories 578 Kc • Protein 43 Gm • Fat 21 Gm • Percent of calories from fat 33% • Cholesterol 99 mg • Dietary Fiber 3 Gm • Sodium 386 mg • Calcium 120 mg

# Warm Lentils and Corn with Lemon Vinaigrette

*Lentils, corn, and radicchio—great color and taste.*

1 cup dried lentils
1 package (1½ teaspoons) onion bouillon
1 cup fresh or frozen corn kernels
¼ cup hazelnut or other nut oil
¼ cup fresh lemon juice
¼ teaspoon salt
2 cups shredded radicchio

½ cup cherry tomatoes, quartered
3 scallions, sliced
1 rib celery, diced
¼ cup chopped fresh flat-leaf parsley
Radicchio leaves for garnish, optional

1. Rinse the lentils and discard any pebbles or stones.

2. Combine the lentils, bouillon, and 2 cups of water in a medium saucepan; bring to a boil over medium heat. Reduce the heat, cover, and simmer 25 to 35 minutes until tender, adding more water if necessary. Add the corn during the last 5 minutes of cooking. Drain.

3. To prepare the vinaigrette, whisk the oil, lemon juice, and salt together in a small saucepan over low heat until warm.

4. Spoon the lentils and corn into a serving bowl. Add the radicchio, tomatoes, scallions, celery, and parsley. Pour the warm dressing over the salad and toss. Garnish with radicchio and serve immediately.

SERVES 4

Kilocalories 337 Kc • Protein 16 Gm • Fat 14 Gm • Percent of calories from fat 36% • Cholesterol 0 mg • Dietary Fiber 16 G • Sodium 421 mg • Calcium 44 mg

# Wild Rice, Basmati, and Escarole Pilaf

*A hint of orange flavor makes this a perfect dish to serve with duck.*

2 tablespoons olive oil
2 medium carrots, diced
1 medium onion, finely chopped
½ cup wild rice
½ cup basmati rice

1 can (13¾ ounces) chicken broth
2 cups chopped escarole
¼ cup chopped pecans
2 teaspoons grated orange
zest

1. Heat the oil over high heat in a Dutch oven; add the carrots and onion and cook 5 minutes, stirring constantly.

2. Add the wild and basmati rice to the pan; cook 1 minute, stirring constantly.

3. Add the broth and place the escarole on top; do not stir. Add 2 cups water; bring to a boil. Cover, reduce the heat, and simmer 45 to 55 minutes, until the rice is done, but chewy.

4. Remove the pot from the heat; stir in the pecans and orange peel; let the pilaf stand, covered, 10 minutes before serving.

SERVES 4

Kilocalories 317 Kc • Protein 7 G • Fat 13 Gm • Percent of calories from fat 36%
• Cholesterol 2 mg • Dietary Fiber 5 Gm • Sodium 58 mg • Calcium 35 mg

# Shrimp and Arugula Risotto

1½ tablespoons olive oil
1 pound medium shrimp, shelled,
    deveined, and cut into thirds
½ teaspoon salt
½ cup dry white wine or bottled
    clam juice

2 cups chicken broth
½ cup minced onion
½ cup diced red bell pepper
1⅓ cups arborio rice
1 bunch arugula, trimmed and
    slivered (about 5 cups)

1. Heat ½ tablespoon of the oil in a Dutch oven or large, heavy saucepan over a medium-high heat. Stir in the shrimp and salt. Cook 1 minute or until the shrimp are pink. Add the wine and cook 2 minutes longer. Remove the shrimp with a slotted spoon; cover with foil and keep warm.

2. Add the broth and 2 cups water to a medium saucepan. Place over low heat, just under a simmer.

3. Heat the remaining 1 tablespoon oil in the Dutch oven over medium heat. Stir in the onion and bell pepper. Cover and cook 5 minutes or until the vegetables are soft. Add the rice, stirring to coat.

4. Add about ½ cup of the hot broth mixture to the rice. Cook, stirring constantly, until the liquid is absorbed, about 5 minutes. Repeat, adding ½ cup broth at a time, until the rice is just tender and creamy, 20 to 25 minutes. Stir in the reserved shrimp and arugula. Cook 2 minutes longer to heat through.

SERVES 4

Kilocalories 477 Kc • Protein 31 Gm • Fat 7 Gm • Percent of calories from fat 13% • Cholesterol 2 mg • Dietary Fiber 2 Gm • Sodium 1427 mg • Calcium 140 mg

# Peppers Stuffed with Bulgur and Broccoli

¼ cup bulgur wheat
1 bunch (about 1 pound) broccoli raab
2 tablespoons plain dried bread crumbs

2 tablespoons grated Romano cheese
1½ tablespoons canola oil
¼ teaspoon salt
2 large red bell peppers, cut in half and seeded

1. Preheat the oven to 400°. Coat a 9-inch square baking pan with vegetable oil spray.

2. Soak the bulgur in 1 cup of hot water for 15 minutes. Drain.

3. Rinse and trim the broccoli raab; cut off the stems from the end to where the leaves begin. (Save the stems for the recipe variation following this one). Chop the leaves and place in a collapsible steamer basket set over simmering water in a wide saucepan. Cover and steam until tender, about 8 minutes. Carefully lift the steamer basket from the saucepan with a long-handled fork and place in the sink. Cool slightly.

4. Combine the broccoli raab with the bulgur, bread crumbs, cheese, 1 tablespoon of the oil, and salt in a medium bowl. Stuff each pepper with the mixture and drizzle with the remaining ½ tablespoon oil. Cover with foil and bake 15 minutes. Uncover and bake 10 minutes longer.

SERVES 4

**Variation:** Cut the broccoli raab stems into 1-inch pieces. Heat 1 tablespoon peanut oil in a wok or skillet over high heat. Add the stems and cook 2 minutes. Add 1 cup julienne of red bell pepper and cook 3 minutes longer, stirring frequently. Splash with 1 tablespoon low-sodium soy sauce and remove from the heat. Serve immediately.

**Kilocalories 143 Kc • Protein 4 Gm • Fat 7 Gm • Percent of calories from fat 40% • Cholesterol 3 mg • Dietary Fiber 6 Gm • Sodium 251 mg • Calcium 204 mg**

# Garlicky Groats and Greens

*This recipe calls for oat groats. Groats are the result of hulling the grain, then crushing it. They're chewy and flavorful.*

2 tablespoons olive oil
2 ribs celery, finely chopped
4 large garlic cloves, minced
2 cups oat groats, rinsed and
   drained

4 cups chopped greens (your
   choice)
½ teaspoon salt
¼ teaspoon freshly ground
   pepper

1. Heat the oil over medium-high heat in a Dutch oven. Sauté the celery and garlic about 3 minutes, stirring frequently, until the celery is softened.

2. Add the groats and sauté 5 minutes, stirring frequently, until lightly browned.

3. Add 5 cups of water and bring to a boil. Reduce the heat, cover, and simmer 40 minutes. Stir in the greens, cover, and cook 5 minutes longer or until the greens are tender. Season with the salt and pepper.

SERVES 6

Kilocalories 237 Kc • Protein 7 G • Fat 6 G • Percent of calories from fat 22% • Cholesterol 0 mg • Dietary Fiber 0 Gm • Sodium 215 mg • Calcium 40 mg

# Quinoa, Mustard Greens, and Dried Cherries

*Quinoa, a gift from the Incas and South America, is the only grain that is considered a complete protein—a vegetarian's dream. It's also an inexpensive source of protein since it expands to four times its dry volume when cooked.*

1 cup quinoa
½ cup dried cherries
2 cups finely chopped fresh
  mustard greens
2 cups drained canned plum
  tomatoes, chopped

1 tablespoon pignoli nuts
½ teaspoon salt
¼ teaspoon freshly ground pepper

1. Rinse the quinoa in a fine-mesh strainer and drain. Combine with 2 cups water in a medium saucepan and bring to a boil.

2. Reduce the heat, add the cherries and simmer, covered, 5 minutes. Top with the greens (do not stir) and cook 5 to 10 minutes longer or until the water has been absorbed.

3. Remove from the heat and stir in the tomatoes, nuts, salt, and pepper. Serve immediately.

SERVES 4

Kilocalories 264 Kc • Protein 9 Gm • Fat 4 Gm • Percent of calories from fat 13% • Cholesterol 0 mg • Dietary Fiber 4 Gm • Sodium 630 mg • Calcium 98 mg

# Groats and Red Chard

*Red Swiss chard adds great color to this dish, but if it is unavailable green Swiss chard may be substituted.*

1 cup oat groats, rinsed and drained
2 tablespoons olive oil
3 garlic cloves, minced
1 bunch (about 1 pound) red Swiss chard, chopped

3 tablespoons chopped fresh flat-leaf parsley
1 tablespoon fresh lemon juice
½ teaspoon salt
¼ cup grated Romano cheese

1. Bring 2 cups of water to a boil in a medium saucepan over high heat. Stir in the groats. Reduce the heat, cover, and simmer about 45 minutes until tender, stirring occasionally.

2. Heat the oil in a large nonstick skillet over medium heat. Add the garlic and cook 2 minutes until lightly browned, stirring frequently.

3. Carefully, add the wet chard. Reduce the heat, cover, and cook about 15 minutes until tender, stirring occasionally.

4. Remove the skillet from the heat; add the parsley, lemon juice, salt, and cooked groats, stirring to combine. Serve sprinkled with the cheese.

SERVES 4

Kilocalories 325 Kc • Protein 17 Gm • Fat 12 Gm • Percent of calories from fat 30% • Cholesterol 6 mg • Dietary Fiber 14 Gm • Sodium 1096 mg • Calcium 327 mg

# Bulgur with Mustard Greens and Dried Fruit (Microwave)

1 cup bulgur wheat
4 cups chopped fresh mustard
   greens
12 dried apricot halves, chopped

¼ cup currants
1 teaspoon caraway seeds
¼ teaspoon ground
   cardamom

1. Combine the bulgur with 2 cups of water in a 3-quart microwave-safe casserole. Cover and microwave on High for 5 minutes; stir. Add the greens, apricots, currants, caraway, and cardamom, stirring to combine. Cover and microwave on Medium for 6 to 8 minutes, until the liquid is absorbed.

2. Let the dish stand 5 minutes and serve.

SERVES 4

Kilocalories 225 Kc • Protein 7 Gm • Fat 1 Gm • Percent of calories from fat 3% • Cholesterol 0 mg • Dietary Fiber 11 Gm • Sodium 19 mg • Calcium 77 mg

# Vegetable and Lollo Rossa Lettuce Rice Salad

*This is a great party salad. It can sit on a buffet for a few hours, if it lasts that long. I prefer the rice slightly undercooked rather than mushy.*

*Salad:*

- 12 cups cooked rice (about 4 cups raw)
- 4 cups julienne of washed Lollo Rossa lettuce (red oak or red leaf lettuce)
- 1 yellow bell pepper, seeded and diced
- 1 cup fresh or frozen (thawed) peas
- ½ cup thinly sliced red onion
- ½ cup chopped fennel
- ¼ cup toasted pumpkin seeds or chopped almonds

*Dressing:*

- ½ cup extra-virgin olive oil
- ½ cup cranberry or red wine vinegar
- 2 tablespoons Dijon mustard
- 1 teaspoon sugar
- 1 teaspoon salt
- ½ teaspoon freshly ground pepper
- ½ teaspoon dried tarragon

1. Combine the rice and 1 cup of the lettuce in a large mixing bowl. Set the remaining lettuce aside.

2. Add the remaining salad ingredients to the bowl, stirring to combine.

3. Whisk all of the dressing ingredients together with ½ cup water in a 2-cup measure. Pour the dressing over the salad mixture and toss. Spoon the salad onto a serving platter. Garnish the rim of the platter with the remaining lettuce.

SERVES 12

**Variation:** Add 1 cup raisins and ½ cup chopped cilantro to the rice salad. Omit the tarragon in the dressing.

Kilocalories 373 Kc • Protein 7 Gm • Fat 12 Gm • Percent of calories from fat 29% • Cholesterol 0 mg • Dietary Fiber 2 Gm • Sodium 214 mg • Calcium 32 mg

# Mini Frittata

*This is a great vegetarian side dish served with steamed vegetables. For brunch, top with julienne of smoked salmon and fresh basil.*

½ cup bulgur wheat
1 tablespoon olive oil
2 cups finely chopped chicory
3 large eggs
½ cup egg substitute or 3 large
   egg whites
⅓ cup grated Romano cheese

¼ cup chopped fresh basil
   (4 teaspoons dried)
¼ teaspoon salt
¼ teaspoon freshly ground
   pepper
Fresh basil  sprigs for garnish

1. Bring 2 cups of water to a boil in a small saucepan. Add the bulgur and cook 5 minutes. Cover and remove from the heat. Let the pan stand 15 minutes; drain well.

2. Heat the oil in a large nonstick skillet over medium heat. Add the chicory, and cook about 5 minutes until wilted and tender, stirring occasionally. Remove from the skillet and cool. Wipe out the skillet.

3. Whisk the eggs, egg substitute, cheese, basil, salt, and pepper together in a large bowl. Stir in the chicory and bulgur.

4. Coat the skillet with vegetable oil spray. Place over medium-low heat. Drop ¼ cupfuls of the egg mixture on the skillet a few inches apart. You probably can fit 3 per batch. Press down with a spatula and cook about 2 minutes or until the edges are set. Turn and cook 1 minute longer. Serve hot or at room temperature. Garnish with basil.

SERVES 4

Kilocalories 230 Kc • Protein 15 Gm • Fat 11 Gm • Percent of calories from fat 42% • Cholesterol 168 mg • Dietary Fiber 7 Gm • Sodium 404 mg • Calcium 218 mg

# Wild Rice, Kale, and Oat Pilaf

*Toasted oats are very flavorful and a great way to add soluble fiber to your diet.*

¾ cup rolled oats
2 tablespoons olive oil
2 medium carrots, diced
½ cup chopped onion
½ cup wild rice

1 can (13¾ ounces) vegetable broth
3 cups chopped kale
2 teaspoons grated orange zest

1. Toast the oats in a Dutch oven over medium heat 5 to 7 minutes, stirring frequently, until lightly browned. Remove the oats and set aside.

2. In the same pan, heat the oil over high heat. Sauté the carrots and onion 5 minutes, stirring constantly. Add the wild rice; cook 1 minute more, stirring constantly.

3. Add the broth, kale, and 1 cup water; bring to a boil. Reduce the heat, cover, and simmer 45 to 55 minutes until cooked but chewy. Remove from the heat; stir in the oats and zest. Let the pot stand, covered, for 10 minutes. Serve.

SERVES 4

Kilocalories 268 Kc • Protein 7 Gm • Fat 8 Gm • Percent of calories from fat 26% • Cholesterol 0 mg • Dietary Fiber 5 Gm • Sodium 64 mg • Calcium 69 mg

# Millet Pilaf with Kohlrabi Greens and Dried Apricots (Pressure Cooker)

*If you like a stickier pilaf, cook an additional 4 minutes at high pressure.*

1½ cups millet (about 10 ounces), rinsed and checked for stones
2 tablespoons vegetable oil
1 medium leek, thinly sliced (white part only)
2 medium carrots, shredded
2 ribs celery, diced
3½ cups vegetable broth or water

1 bunch kohlrabi greens, chopped (about 8 cups)
½ cup chopped dried apricots or other dried fruit
¼ teaspoon ground allspice
Salt
¼ cup slivered almonds for garnish, optional

1. Toast the millet in the open pressure cooker over high heat, stirring frequently, until the millet starts to pop and becomes fragrant, 4 to 5 minutes. Add the oil and stir to coat. Stir in the leek, carrots, and celery and cook 1 minute, stirring constantly. Add the broth, greens, apricots, allspice, and salt to taste.

2. Lock the lid in place and bring to high pressure over high heat. Adjust the heat to maintain high pressure; cook 16 minutes. Let the pressure drop naturally for 10 minutes before removing the lid. Remove the lid, tilting it away from you to allow the excess steam to escape.

3. Serve immediately and garnish with the almonds, if desired.

SERVES 6

Kilocalories 309 Kc • Protein 8 Gm • Fat 7 Gm • Percent of calories from fat 19% • Cholesterol 0 mg • Dietary Fiber 8 Gm • Sodium 84 mg • Calcium 75 mg

# Spanish-Style Chicken, Greens, and Rice (Microwave)

*Converted rice is rice that has been parboiled before packaging. It's a method for retaining nutrients yet yielding a rice that is firm-textured and separate when cooked.*

1 cup chopped onion
½ cup chopped green bell pepper
2 teaspoons vegetable oil
2 garlic cloves, minced
2 cups (16-ounce can) whole peeled tomatoes
2 cups chopped tat soi or spinach
2 tablespoons chopped fresh flat-leaf parsley
1 teaspoon dried oregano

½ teaspoon salt
¼ teaspoon ground cumin
¼ teaspoon freshly ground pepper
1 bay leaf
4 ounces long-grain converted rice
1 (3-pound) chicken, cut into 8 pieces and skinned
8 pimiento-stuffed olives, sliced

1. Combine the onion, green pepper, oil, and garlic in a 3-quart microwave-safe bowl. Cover with wax paper or a vented cover and microwave on High for 2 minutes. Stir in the tomatoes with their juice, greens, parsley, oregano, salt, cumin, pepper, and bay leaf. Cover and cook on High for 2 minutes, or until the mixture comes to a boil.

2. Stir in the rice. Cover and cook on Medium-high for 7 minutes. Add the chicken pieces, pushing them down into the rice. Cover and cook on Medium-high for 10 minutes. Stir, cover, and cook 6 minutes longer. Stir in the olives and let the pot stand for 10 minutes. Discard the bay leaf before serving.

SERVES 4

Kilocalories 737 Kc • Protein 97 Gm • Fat 27 Gm • Percent of calories from fat 34% • Cholesterol 282 mg • Dietary Fiber 3 Gm • Sodium 924 mg • Calcium 139 mg

# Brown Basmati Rice with Dandelion and Elephant Garlic (Pressure Cooker)

*Oversized elephant garlic tastes more like a strong-flavored leek than garlic. If you can't find this ingredient you can substitute leeks or regular onions.*

1 package (16 ounces) dried kidney beans
1 tablespoon vegetable oil
¾ cup chopped elephant garlic (about 3 large bulbs)
1 cup brown basmati rice (or regular brown rice)
7 cups vegetable broth or water

1 bunch dandelion greens (about 1¼ pounds), trimmed and coarsely chopped
1 small jalapeño pepper, seeded and chopped (¼ teaspoon Tabasco sauce)
¼ cup chopped fresh flat-leaf parsley
Salt

1. Soak the beans in water overnight or use the quick-soak method (page 240).

2. Heat the oil in an open pressure cooker over medium heat; add the elephant garlic and cook 1 minute, stirring frequently. Stir in the rice to coat. Add the broth, greens, jalapeño, and drained beans. Lock the lid in place and bring to high pressure over high heat. Adjust the heat to maintain high pressure and cook 10 minutes. Let the pressure drop naturally for 10 minutes. Open the lid, tilting it away from you to allow the excess steam to escape.

3. Stir in the parsley and season to taste with salt.

SERVES 6

Kilocalories 492 Kc • Protein 25 Gm • Fat 5 Gm • Percent of calories from fat 9% • Cholesterol 0 mg • Dietary Fiber 25 Gm • Sodium 226 mg • Calcium 333 mg

# Pecan Rice Salad and Radicchio

*Great with chicken, duck, or quail.*

1 cup long-grain rice
⅓ cup fresh orange juice
2 tablespoons chopped fresh flat-leaf parsley
2 tablespoons apple cider vinegar
1 tablespoon olive oil
1 tablespoon minced shallots

2 teaspoons honey
1 teaspoon grated orange zest
⅛ teaspoon salt
2 small seedless oranges, peeled and cut in 1-inch pieces
1 cup finely chopped radicchio
2 tablespoons chopped pecans

1. Bring 2 cups of water to a boil in a medium saucepan. Stir in the rice; cover, and reduce the heat. Simmer 20 minutes, until the water is absorbed and the rice is tender. Place in a serving bowl.

2. While the rice is cooking, whisk the juice, parsley, vinegar, oil, shallots, honey, zest, and salt together in a 1-cup measure. Pour over the rice in the bowl and toss to coat. Stir in the oranges, radicchio, and pecans. Serve warm or at room temperature.

SERVES 4

Kilocalories 276 Kc • Protein 5 Gm • Fat 6 Gm • Percent of calories from fat 19%
• Cholesterol 0 mg • Dietary Fiber 3 Gm • Sodium 79 mg • Calcium 49 mg

# Brown Rice and Napa Cabbage
# with Warm Vinaigrette

*This is a main-dish vegetarian salad.*

3 cups finely shredded napa or
   Chinese cabbage
1½ cups cooked and cooled
   brown rice
1 cup coarsely shredded carrot
½ cup thinly sliced scallions, cut
   on diagonal

*Dressing:*

3 tablespoons rice wine vinegar
1½ tablespoons vegetable oil

1 tablespoon water
1 tablespoon reduced-sodium
   soy sauce
1 teaspoon dark sesame oil
1 garlic clove, crushed through a
   press
1 teaspoon grated fresh ginger
½ teaspoon salt
1 tablespoon toasted sesame
   seeds for garnish, optional

1. Combine the cabbage, rice, carrot, and scallions in a large serving bowl.

2. Whisk all of the dressing ingredients together in a small saucepan. Bring to a simmer over low heat. Pour the warm dressing over the salad and toss to coat. Sprinkle with the sesame seeds, if desired.

SERVES 4

Kilocalories 181 Kc • Protein 4 Gm • Fat 7 Gm • Percent of calories from fat 36%
• Cholesterol 0 mg • Dietary Fiber 4 Gm • Sodium 474 mg • Calcium 47 mg

# Quinoa- and Spinach-Stuffed Turkey Breast

*Although crisp roasted poultry skin looks and tastes great, it's wise to remove the skin before eating the turkey to significantly reduce its fat content.*

½ cup quinoa
1 tablespoon vegetable oil
1 cup finely chopped stemmed shiitake mushrooms
½ cup (packed) baby spinach or mache, plus additional for garnish, optional
¼ cup chopped pimiento
1 tablespoon chopped fresh flat-leaf parsley

1 tablespoon chopped fresh tarragon (1 teaspoon dried)
½ teaspoon salt
2 pounds (approximately) boneless turkey breast, in one piece
¼ teaspoon freshly ground pepper
½ teaspoon paprika

1. Preheat the oven to 350°.

2. To prepare the stuffing, rinse the quinoa in a fine-mesh strainer and drain. Combine with 1 cup water in a medium saucepan and bring to a boil. Reduce the heat and simmer, covered, 10 to 15 minutes or until all the water is absorbed.

3. Heat the oil in a large nonstick skillet over medium heat. Add the mushrooms and cook about 5 minutes, until soft, stirring occasionally. Add the baby spinach and cook 2 minutes longer. Stir the cooked quinoa, pimiento, parsley, tarragon, and salt into the skillet. Cook 2 minutes and set aside.

4. Rinse the turkey and pat it dry with paper towels. Place it skin side down on wax paper. Cut across through the thickest part to within 1 inch of the end and open like a book. Cover with wax paper and pound with a meat mallet to a ½-inch thickness, making a rectangle about 8 × 16 inches. Sprinkle with the pepper.

5. Spoon the stuffing down the center to within 1 inch of the ends. Lift one long edge over the filling and secure to the other long edge with toothpicks. Place on a 15 × 10-inch jelly roll pan, skin side up. Sprinkle with the paprika.

6. Roast 35 minutes or until the juices run clear when the meat is pricked with a fork, and a meat thermometer registers 170°. Let the turkey stand for 10 minutes before slicing it. Place the slices on a serving platter and garnish the rim of the platter with baby spinach or mache, if desired.

SERVES 6

Kilocalories 293 Kc • Protein 48 Gm • Fat 4 Gm • Percent of calories from fat 14% • Cholesterol 126 mg • Dietary Fiber 2 Gm • Sodium 87 mg • Calcium 35 mg

# Mushroom, Spinach, and Wheat Berry Salad

*Much of this salad can be prepared ahead of time. Cook the wheat berries and rice early in the day and make and refrigerate the dressing up to a day before. Prepare the salad 30 minutes before serving. It's great for summer entertaining.*

½ cup wheat berries

*Dressing:*

½ cup fresh lemon juice
3 tablespoons olive oil
1 teaspoon Dijon mustard
1 garlic clove, crushed through a press
½ teaspoon salt
½ teaspoon sugar
¼ teaspoon freshly ground pepper

*Salad:*

1 cup thin slices small white mushrooms
4 cups (packed) chopped fresh spinach
2 cups cooked and cooled white rice
½ cup thinly sliced red onion
½ cup halved seedless red grapes
⅓ cup slivered smoked turkey ham (about 2 ounces), optional

1. Soak the wheat berries in cold water overnight. Drain and rinse the wheat berries and place them in a large saucepan with 2 quarts water. Bring to a boil over high heat, stirring occasionally. Reduce the heat and simmer about 45 minutes until the wheat is puffed and tender. Drain and cool.

2. Whisk all of the dressing ingredients together with 2 tablespoons water in a large serving bowl. Stir in the mushrooms and let the mixture stand at room temperature 30 minutes.

3. Add the wheat berries, spinach, rice, onion, grapes, and ham, if desired. Toss and serve.

SERVES 4

Kilocalories 329 Kc • Protein 8 Gm • Fat 11 Gm • Percent of calories from fat 30% • Cholesterol 0 mg • Dietary Fiber 3 Gm • Sodium 345 mg • Calcium 80 mg

# Chilean Corn Casserole

2 teaspoons vegetable oil
1 cup chopped onion
2 large garlic cloves, minced
1 pound chicken or meatless
  sausage, cut into 1-inch pieces
4 cups chopped collard greens
¼ cup golden raisins

1 can (15 ounces) creamed
  corn
1 hard-cooked egg,
  chopped
1 hard-cooked egg white,
  chopped
1 teaspoon sugar

1. Preheat the oven to 350°.

2. Combine the oil, onion, and garlic in a large nonstick skillet over medium heat. Cover and cook 3 minutes, stirring occasionally, until soft.

3. Add the sausage and cook, stirring frequently, until no longer pink, about 5 minutes.

4. Top with the wet collards, raisins, and 2 tablespoons water. Cover and cook 5 minutes until the collards are wilted and the raisins are plumped.

5. Remove from the heat and stir in the corn, egg, and egg white. Spoon the sausage mixture into a 1½-quart casserole coated with vegetable oil spray. Sprinkle with the sugar and bake 30 minutes until lightly browned and bubbly. Let the casserole stand 10 minutes before serving.

SERVES 3

Kilocalories 489 Kc • Protein 40 Gm • Fat 22 Gm • Percent of calories from fat 37%
• Cholesterol 151 mg • Dietary Fiber 10 Gm • Sodium 1361 mg • Calcium 541 mg

# Whole Wheat Couscous with Broccoli Raab and Raisins

*Technically couscous is a pasta made from finely ground durum wheat. The whole wheat variety is made from coarsely ground durum wheat and is treated as a grain. I often serve this as a main-dish meal.*

1½ tablespoons olive oil
1 bunch broccoli raab (about 1¼ pounds), trimmed and coarsely chopped (wet)

½ cup dark raisins
½ teaspoon salt
1 cup whole wheat couscous

1. Heat 1 tablespoon of the oil in a large nonstick skillet over medium heat. Add the broccoli raab, raisins, and salt. Cover and cook, stirring frequently, 10 minutes.

2. While the broccoli raab is cooking, bring 2 cups water to a boil in a medium, heavy-bottomed saucepan. Stir in the couscous and reduce the heat. Cover and simmer 5 minutes, until the water is absorbed. Stir into the broccoli raab mixture and drizzle with the remaining ½ tablespoon oil. Serve immediately.

SERVES 4

Kilocalories 307 Kc • Protein 7 Gm • Fat 5 Gm • Percent of calories from fat 15% • Cholesterol 0 mg • Dietary Fiber 10 Gm • Sodium 344 mg • Calcium 203 mg

# Skillet Brown Rice and Vegetables

*Don't be fooled by the amount of ingredients in this recipe. It's really a very simple dish to make.*

1 cup brown rice
1 cup thinly sliced celery
1 cup chopped green bell pepper
1 cup cooked chopped greens
   (mustard, turnip, collard)
½ cup sliced scallions
¼ cup dark raisins
2 cups coarsely grated low-fat
   Monterey Jack cheese (about 8
   ounces)

½ ounce cashews, chopped
2 tablespoons vegetable oil
2 tablespoons vegetable broth
   or water
1 tablespoon sesame seeds
1 tablespoon sunflower
   seeds
1 teaspoon mixed herb salt-free
   seasoning
6 plum tomatoes, cut into
   wedges

1. Cook the rice according to the package directions. Drain.

2. Combine the rice with the remaining ingredients except the tomatoes and ½ cup of the cheese in a large nonstick skillet. Top with the tomatoes and sprinkle with the reserved cheese. Cover and cook over low heat just until heated through, about 15 minutes.

SERVES 4

Kilocalories 502 Kc • Protein 23 Gm • Fat 25 Gm • Percent of calories from fat 42%
• Cholesterol 40 mg • Dietary Fiber 4 Gm • Sodium 617 mg • Calcium 91 mg

# 7
# Greens and Beans

Legumes are podded seeds. They are a good source of protein and include not only beans, but also peas, lentils, and peanuts.

Dried beans are very economical. One cup yields 3 to 3½ cups cooked beans and they may be frozen after they are cooked. They are a great meat substitute—allow 2 ounces of beans for every ounce of meat.

If you don't have time to soak and cook beans, use canned ones. They're great in a pinch. Canned beans come in two sizes: 15 ounces and 19 ounces. Each bean yields a different cup measure because of its size and shape. The drained amount in each can ranges from 1¾ cups to 2⅛ cups. A good rule of thumb is to assume that either size can will yield about 2 cups of cooked beans.

Heirloom beans are varieties grown from old seed stock. These beans are quite exotic and are only grown in small quantities. A few recipes in this chapter use heirloom beans. They can be purchased in specialty food shops and health food stores.

Because they have no fat or cholesterol, "Beans, beans are good for your heart . . ."—we all know the ending to that rhyme. Fortunately, we can eliminate the gaseous effects of beans by soaking them before cooking. You may use any of the following methods:

1. *Overnight soak*: Place the beans in a large pot and pour in cold water to cover by 2 inches. Let the pot stand overnight. Drain.
2. *Quick-boil soak*: Cover the beans with cold water. Bring to a boil for 2 minutes. Remove from the heat. Cover the pot and let it stand 1 hour. Drain.
3. *Hot-soak method*: Pour boiling water over the beans in the pot. Let them stand 1 hour. Drain.

Tips for cooking beans:

1. Do not add salt, baking soda, or acidic ingredients like tomatoes, wine, or fruit juices to the simmering beans. These ingredients will toughen the skins and make the beans less palatable.
2. Fat added to simmering water will reduce the foaming while the beans are cooking, but it's not necessary. If foam rises to the top of the pot, just skim it off with a spoon.

# Beans and Greens Chili

*I add a bunch of broccoli raab to this delicious vegetarian chili. I include most of the stem, but if you prefer to use just leaves and buds, add two bunches of this green. Serve with a potful of brown rice and crusty bread to sop up the juices.*

1 cup chopped onion
1 small fennel bulb, chopped (about 2 cups)
3 ribs celery, chopped
2 tablespoons vegetable oil
3 garlic cloves, minced
2 tablespoons crushed cumin seed
1 can (28 ounces) Italian-style tomatoes with juice
12 ounces light beer
3 tablespoons chili powder
1 tablespoon dried oregano (3 tablespoons fresh)
1 teaspoon salt
1 teaspoon freshly ground pepper
1 cup cooked chickpeas
1 cup cooked kidney beans
1 cup cooked corn kernels
1 bunch broccoli raab, trimmed and coarsely chopped
½ cup snipped fresh dill

1. Combine the onion, fennel, celery, oil, garlic, and cumin in a Dutch oven. Cover and cook over low heat for 15 minutes, stirring occasionally, until the vegetables are tender.

2. Coarsely chop the tomatoes in the can with a scissors; add to the Dutch oven with the beer, chili powder, oregano, salt, and pepper. Cook, covered, 30 minutes, stirring occasionally.

3. Stir in the chickpeas, kidney beans, and corn and top with the wet broccoli raab; cook 30 minutes longer, stirring occasionally. Stir in the dill and serve immediately.

SERVES 6

Kilocalories 240 Kc • Protein 8 Gm • Fat 7 Gm • Percent of calories from fat 24% • Cholesterol 0 mg • Dietary Fiber 8 Gm • Sodium 1070 mg • Calcium 158 mg

# Spinach and Bean Soufflé

*Soufflés are puffed egg-based dishes that may be savory or sweet. This light and airy greens and beans soufflé may be served as a main dish with a salad and a warm, herbed grain side dish.*

1 cup cooked beans (kidney, cannellini, or navy beans)
1 package (10 ounces) frozen chopped spinach, thawed, drained, and squeezed
1 cup 1% milk
2 tablespoons cornstarch
5 large eggs, separated (discard 1 yolk)

1 tablespoon (packed) dark brown sugar
½ teaspoon salt
¼ teaspoon grated nutmeg
¼ teaspoon freshly ground pepper
¼ teaspoon cream of tartar

1. Preheat the oven to 375°.

2. Combine the beans and spinach in a food processor fitted with a steel blade. Process until the mixture is smooth.

3. Whisk the milk, cornstarch, egg yolks, sugar, salt, nutmeg, and pepper together in a 2-cup measure. Pour over the bean mixture in the food processor. Process until combined, about 20 seconds. Transfer the mixture to a large bowl.

4. Beat the egg whites in a large bowl of an electric mixer at medium-low speed until frothy. Add the cream of tartar and beat at medium-high speed until stiff, but not dry, peaks form. Gently fold a little at a time into the bean mixture until all of the white streaks are completely blended. Spoon the mixture into a 6-cup soufflé dish coated with vegetable oil spray. Place the dish in a 13 × 9-inch baking pan; place on an oven rack. Pour boiling water into the baking pan to come halfway up the side of the soufflé dish. Bake 50 minutes, until puffed and browned. Serve immediately.

SERVES 6

Kilocalories 162 Kc • Protein 11 Gm • Fat 5 Gm • Percent of calories from fat 26%
• Cholesterol 178 mg • Dietary Fiber 4 Gm • Sodium 504 mg • Calcium 163 mg

# Chicory, Turnip, and Lentil Gratin

*This hearty winter dish can double as a main course, especially if you substitute sliced potatoes for the turnips.*

1 cup vegetable or chicken broth
1 cup lentils, picked over and
    washed
1 bunch chicory (about 12
    ounces), trimmed and chopped
½ cup plain dried bread
    crumbs
¼ cup oat bran
3 medium turnips (about 1 pound),
    pared and thinly sliced

¾ teaspoon salt
1 tablespoon vegetable oil
1 can (12 ounces) evaporated
    skimmed milk
1 cup shredded Gruyère cheese
    or Swiss cheese (about
    4 ounces)
½ teaspoon paprika

1. Preheat the oven to 375°.

2. Combine the broth with 2 cups water; bring to a boil in a medium saucepan. Add the lentils, reduce the heat, cover, and simmer 15 minutes. Place the chicory on top of the lentils in the pan, pushing down to fit. Cover and cook 10 minutes longer. Drain in a large colander; stir to combine.

3. Combine the bread crumbs and oat bran in a small bowl.

4. Layer half of the chicory mixture in an 11 × 7-inch baking dish coated with vegetable oil spray; top with all of the turnips. Sprinkle with ½ teaspoon of the salt and half of the bread crumb mixture. Arrange the remaining chicory mixture over the turnips and sprinkle with the remaining ¼ teaspoon salt and the rest of the bread crumb mixture; drizzle with the oil. Pour the milk over all; sprinkle the cheese and paprika over the top.

5. Cover with foil and bake 30 minutes. Remove the foil and bake 15 to 20 minutes longer or until lightly browned and tender. Let the dish stand 5 minutes before serving.

SERVES 4

**Kilocalories 481 Kc • Protein 33 Gm • Fat 15 Gm • Percent of calories from fat 26%**
**• Cholesterol 35 mg • Dietary Fiber 22 Gm • Sodium 823 mg • Calcium 687 mg**

# Molasses Baked Beans and Greens

*Lima beans are used instead of the traditional navy bean. This recipe calls for the addition of salt at the beginning of baking. It won't affect the texture of the beans because of the slow-cooking method. This rich, syrupy winter dish will fill your home with a fabulous aroma.*

2 cups dried lima beans
½ cup chopped onion
½ cup molasses
¼ cup (packed) brown
  sugar

2 teaspoons dry mustard
1 teaspoon salt
8 cups coarsely chopped Swiss
  chard or collard greens

1. Use the overnight or quick-soaking method for the beans (page 240); drain.

2. Preheat the oven to 350°.

3. Combine the beans, onion, and 10 cups of water in a large Dutch oven.

4. Combine the molasses, sugar, mustard, and salt in a small bowl; stir into the bean mixture. Cover and bake 3 hours, stirring occasionally.

5. Stir in the greens, cover, and bake an additional hour. Uncover and bake 1½ hours longer until the mixture is thick and syrupy. Serve immediately.

SERVES 8

Kilocalories 251 Kc • Protein 12 Gm • Fat 0 Gm • Percent of calories from fat 2% • Cholesterol 0 mg • Dietary Fiber 11 Gm • Sodium 565 mg • Calcium 260 mg

# Chicory in Bean Purée

*Puréed beans are also delicious and nutritious as a salad dressing.*

1 head chicory (about
   1 pound), steamed, chopped,
   and drained

*Puree:*

2 cups cooked chickpeas
1 tablespoon fresh lemon juice
½ teaspoon salt
¼ teaspoon freshly ground
   pepper

¼ cup chopped fresh flat-leaf
   parsley

*Topping:*

1 tablespoon olive oil
1 cup thinly sliced green bell
   pepper
½ cup thinly sliced onion
⅛ teaspoon salt

1. Preheat the oven to 375°.

2. Place the chicory in an 11 × 7-inch baking dish coated with vegetable oil spray.

3. Combine the chickpeas with ½ cup water, the lemon juice, salt, and pepper in a food processor or blender. Purée until smooth. Stir in the parsley and spoon the mixture over the chicory.

4. Heat the oil in a medium nonstick skillet over medium-high heat. Add the bell pepper and onion and cook, stirring frequently, until lightly browned, about 5 minutes. Spoon the mixture over the beans, sprinkle with the salt, and bake 20 to 25 minutes until heated through.

SERVES 4

Kilocalories 211 Kc • Protein 11 Gm • Fat 6 Gm • Percent of calories from fat 23%
• Cholesterol 0 mg • Dietary Fiber 19 Gm • Sodium 867 mg • Calcium 405 mg

# Soybean Burgers with Cabbage Slaw

*This departure from the venerable hamburger is topped with a cabbage slaw instead of ketchup and pickles.*

8 ounces soybeans (about 1¼ cups)

**Cabbage Slaw:**

2 tablespoons light mayonnaise
2 teaspoons apple cider vinegar
¼ teaspoon salt
¼ teaspoon freshly ground
   pepper
1 cup finely shredded green
   cabbage

½ cup thinly sliced red onion
½ cup shredded carrot

**Burgers:**

1 cup rolled oats
2 large egg whites
2 teaspoons chili powder
½ teaspoon salt
½ teaspoon freshly ground pepper
4 whole wheat burger buns

    1. Soak the beans using your preferred method (page 240).

    2. Combine the beans and 4 cups water in a 3-quart saucepan. Bring to a boil. Reduce the heat and simmer, partially covered, about 3 hours or until tender. Drain.

    3. To prepare the slaw, whisk the mayonnaise, vinegar, salt, and pepper together in a medium bowl. Add the cabbage, onion, and carrot; toss to coat. Refrigerate, covered, until ready to use. Let stand at room temperature 30 minutes before serving.

    4. To prepare the burgers, combine the soybeans, oats, egg whites, chili powder, salt, and pepper in a food processor fitted with the steel blade. Pulse to combine, then process about 30 seconds until smooth, scraping down the sides of the bowl. Fill a 1-cup dry measure with just under ¾ cup of the soybean mixture. Unmold onto wax paper. Repeat with the remaining mixture to make 4 mounds. Shape each mound into a patty.

    5. Coat a large nonstick skillet with vegetable oil spray and place over medium heat. When the skillet is hot, carefully add the patties with a spatula. Cook about 5 minutes on each side until browned. Place each patty on the bottom of a bun; top each with about ½ cup slaw and cover with a top bun. Serve immediately.

SERVES 4

Kilocalories 410 Kc • Protein 26 Gm • Fat 14 Gm • Percent of calories from fat 29%
• Cholesterol 0 mg • Dietary Fiber 10 Gm • Sodium 768 mg • Calcium 177 mg

# Cinnamon Spinach, Pumpkin, and Great Northern Beans

*This dish may be made a day or two before serving. For an intense cinnamon flavor, don't remove the cinnamon stick until after reheating.*

4 cups peeled and cubed (2-inch pieces) pumpkin (1 small pumpkin, about 1½ pounds)
1 (3-inch) cinnamon stick
10 ounces fresh spinach, trimmed

2 cups cooked Great Northern beans (or other white bean)
¼ teaspoon salt
¼ teaspoon freshly ground pepper

Combine the pumpkin and cinnamon stick with 4 cups water in a large saucepan. Bring to a boil over high heat. Cook 12 to 15 minutes until just tender. Reduce the heat to medium, add the spinach, cover, and cook 2 minutes. Top with the beans and cook 2 minutes longer. Stir in the salt and pepper and serve.

SERVES 4

Kilocalories 215 Kc • Protein 13 Gm • Fat 1 Gm • Percent of calories from fat 4%
• Cholesterol 0 mg • Dietary Fiber 9 Gm • Sodium 209 mg • Calcium 181 mg

# Cassoulet

*Cassoulet is traditionally a very high-fat French casserole. You won't find confit of duck or goose, pork or French sausage in this low-fat version, but what you will find is lots of flavor.*

2 cups flageolets (small French kidney beans) or small white beans
4 sprigs fresh flat-leaf parsley
1 tablespoon fresh thyme (2 teaspoons dried)
5 whole peppercorns
3 slices turkey bacon, finely chopped
1 bay leaf
1 medium onion studded with 6 cloves
1 cup diced carrot

1 tablespoon olive oil
8 ounces turkey sausage, sliced
½ cup chopped onion
1 garlic clove, minced
4 cups chopped frisee or collard greens
½ cup tomato puree
½ teaspoon salt
½ teaspoon freshly ground pepper
1 cup fresh bread crumbs

1. Rinse and sort the beans. Soak, according to your preferred method (page 240).

2. Combine the parsley, thyme, and peppercorns in a cheesecloth bag.

3. Drain the beans and add to a Dutch oven with 8 cups of water. Add the bacon, herb bag, bay leaf, onion, and carrot. Bring to a boil. Reduce the heat and simmer, partially covered, 1½ hours. Remove the herb bag, bay leaf, and studded onion.

4. Preheat the oven to 375°.

5. Meanwhile, heat the oil in a medium nonstick skillet over medium heat. Add the turkey sausage and chopped onion; cook 5 minutes, stirring frequently. Add the garlic; cook 30 seconds. Stir in the wet frisee, tomato puree, salt, pepper, and 2 tablespoons water. Cover and cook 2 minutes. Stir into the bean mixture; top with the bread crumbs. Bake, uncovered, 1 hour. Serve immediately.

SERVES 4

Kilocalories 645 Kc • Protein 38 Gm • Fat 13 Gm • Percent of calories from fat 17% • Cholesterol 37 mg • Dietary Fiber 22 Gm • Sodium 1089 mg • Calcium 278 mg

# Chilled Black Bean Casserole

*This is a terrific party dish. It can be made a day or two ahead.*

3 cups thinly sliced onion
2 tablespoons vegetable oil
2 teaspoons sugar
2 bunches watercress, trimmed
  and chopped, *or* 6 cups
  chopped fresh spinach
2 cups cooked black beans

1 cup cooked fresh or frozen
  corn kernels
2 ripe tomatoes, diced
⅓ cup chopped fresh
  cilantro
3 tablespoons apple cider vinegar
2 scallions, thinly sliced
½ teaspoon salt

1. Combine the onion, oil, and sugar in a medium nonstick skillet. Cover and cook over low heat 10 minutes. Uncover, increase the heat to medium and cook 5 to 10 minutes longer, stirring frequently, until lightly browned and caramelized.

2. Combine the onion mixture with all of the remaining ingredients in a serving bowl. Refrigerate, covered, at least 1 hour before serving.

SERVES 6

Kilocalories 189 Kc • Protein 8 Gm • Fat 5 Gm • Percent of calories from fat 24% • Cholesterol 0 mg • Dietary Fiber 8 Gm • Sodium 304 mg • Calcium 79 mg

# Dandelion and Christmas Lima Beans in Phyllo Crust

*This is a deep-dish pie—a savory and slightly more sophisticated version of apple pandowny. Christmas lima beans, an heirloom bean, have a faint chestnut taste. If you can't find them in specialty food stores, use large lima beans.*

1 tablespoon vegetable oil
½ cup chopped onion
6 cups chopped dandelion greens (turnip greens may be substituted)
2 cups cooked Christmas lima beans
1 tablespoon sugar
½ teaspoon salt

3 medium apples (Delicious, Empire, or Cortland)
1 tablespoon fresh lemon juice
6 sheets phyllo dough
1 tablespoon thin lemon zest strips (a zesting tool is best for this)
2 tablespoons all-purpose flour
1 tablespoon unsalted butter, melted

1. Preheat the oven to 350°.

2. Heat the oil in a large nonstick skillet over medium heat. Add the onion and cook 1 minute, stirring frequently, until tender. Add the wet dandelion greens, cover, and cook 3 minutes, stirring once, until wilted. Stir in the beans, sugar, and salt. Remove from the heat.

3. Peel and grate the apples. Place them in a medium bowl and toss with the lemon juice; set aside.

4. Stack the phyllo sheets and cut in half crosswise. Cover with damp paper towels. Coat a 1-quart glass casserole dish with vegetable oil spray. Gently press a half sheet of phyllo into the dish, allowing the ends to extend over the edges of the dish; lightly coat the phyllo with vegetable oil spray. Place another half-sheet of phyllo across the first sheet to form a crisscross design; lightly coat with vegetable oil spray. Repeat with 4 more layers.

5. Spoon the dandelion mixture into the phyllo-lined casserole dish and sprinkle with the lemon zest.

6. Sprinkle the apples with flour and toss to coat; spoon over the dandelion mixture in the dish.

7. To enclose the filling, top the apple mixture with the remaining 6 sheets of phyllo, following the instructions in step 4. Fold in the edges to fit the pan and form a rim. Drizzle the butter on the top layer of phyllo and bake 40 to 45 minutes until golden.

SERVES 4

**Kilocalories 298 Kc • Protein 6 Gm • Fat 10 Gm • Percent of calories from fat 29% • Cholesterol 8 mg • Dietary Fiber 14 Gm • Sodium 509 mg • Calcium 217 mg**

# Mung Bean Stew

*Mung beans, found at ethnic markets and health food stores, are commonly used to grow bean sprouts.*

2 tablespoons vegetable oil
½ teaspoon cumin seeds, crushed
¼ teaspoon ground red pepper
6 ounces yellow split mung beans (unsprouted)
½ cup finely chopped onion
2 garlic cloves, minced
2 teaspoons grated fresh ginger
½ teaspoon ground turmeric

3 cups cauliflower florets
2 cups chopped fresh mustard greens
1 large potato (about 6 ounces), pared and cut into 1-inch cubes
1½ teaspoons salt
2 tablespoons chopped fresh cilantro

Heat the oil in a Dutch oven over medium-high heat. Add the cumin seeds; cook about 30 seconds, until they are dark brown in color. Stir in the red pepper and cook 30 seconds. Add the mung beans, onion, garlic, ginger, turmeric, and 3 cups water to the casserole. Bring to a boil. Reduce the heat and simmer, partially covered, 15 minutes, stirring occasionally. Add the cauliflower, greens, potato, salt, and 1 more cup of water; cook 45 minutes, until the beans and vegetables are tender, stirring frequently. Sprinkle with the cilantro and serve.

SERVES 4

Kilocalories 291 Kc • Protein 15 Gm • Fat 8 Gm • Percent of calories from fat 24% • Cholesterol 0 mg • Dietary Fiber 12 Gm • Sodium 915 mg • Calcium 159 mg

# Escarole, Radicchio, and White Beans

2 teaspoons olive oil
2 cups thinly sliced red onion
1 large garlic clove, minced
2 cups cooked cannellini beans
(19-ounce can)
1 tablespoon fresh sage
(1 teaspoon dried)

6 cups (packed) chopped
escarole
2 cups chopped
radicchio lettuce
¼ teaspoon salt

1. Heat the oil in a Dutch oven over medium heat. Stir in the onion to coat. Cover and cook for 3 minutes. Uncover, add the garlic, and cook 2 minutes, stirring occasionally.

2. Add the beans with their liquid and the sage; cook 5 minutes, stirring occasionally.

3. Stir in the escarole and radicchio; add ½ cup of water and the salt. Cover and cook 5 to 8 minutes longer, stirring once, until the greens are wilted and tender.

SERVES 2

Kilocalories 395 Kc • Protein 22 Gm • Fat 6 Gm • Percent of calories from fat 13%
• Cholesterol 0 mg • Dietary Fiber 19 Gm • Sodium 349 mg • Calcium 326 mg

# Fiddlehead Ferns, Collards, and Black Beans

*Fiddlehead ferns, tightly coiled little green fronds, are available from late March until the end of June in specialty food stores and green-markets. They're what I'd call the pre-leafy greens stage. When they do sprout and become bona fide ferns, they're inedible. So enjoy them while they last.*

2 cups (about 4 ounces) fiddlehead ferns, washed and trimmed

1 package (10 ounces) frozen chopped collard greens, thawed and drained

1 cup cooked black beans

½ cup chopped onion

1 small jalapeño, seeded and minced (or ⅛ teaspoon ground red pepper)

Salt

½ cup shredded Monterey Jack cheese (about 1½ ounces)

1. Preheat the broiler.

2. Cook the ferns with 1 cup water in a medium saucepan over medium heat for 10 minutes. Add the collards, beans, onion, and jalapeño, cover, and cook 5 minutes longer; drain. Season with salt.

3. Place the drained mixture in a gratin dish or 9-inch pie dish and top with the cheese. Broil 2 inches from the heat for about 3 minutes or until browned. Serve immediately.

SERVES 2

Kilocalories 294 Kc • Protein 19 Gm • Fat 10 Gm • Percent of calories from fat 29% • Cholesterol 30 mg • Dietary Fiber 8 Gm • Sodium 497 mg • Calcium 540 mg

# Dandelion and White Beans in Garlic Oil

1 bunch dandelion greens (about 1½ pounds), trimmed and chopped

1 tablespoon extra-virgin olive oil

2 large garlic cloves, minced

2 cups cooked cannellini beans (19-ounce can, drained)

½ teaspoon salt

1. Place the dandelion greens in a collapsible steamer basket set over simmering water in a wide saucepan. Cover and steam 5 minutes until bright green.

2. While the greens are steaming, heat the oil in a large nonstick skillet over medium heat. Add the garlic and cook 30 seconds. Stir in the beans, greens, and salt. Cook 2 minutes longer, until heated through. Serve immediately.

SERVES 4

Kilocalories 302 Kc • Protein 18 Gm • Fat 5 Gm • Percent of calories from fat 15% • Cholesterol 0 mg • Dietary Fiber 18 Gm • Sodium 409 mg • Calcium 474 mg

# Greens and Beans in Two-Tomato Sauce

*Fresh tomatoes and dried tomatoes are a terrific twosome. Combined with heirloom rice beans, which look more like pignoli nuts than rice kernels, this is a very Mediterranean dish. For a main course serve over rice or orzo.*

1 cup rice beans (or other small white bean)

1 head escarole or bunch Swiss chard, trimmed and chopped

½ teaspoon salt

*Sauce:*

1 cup sun-dried tomatoes, soaked in ½ cup boiling water for 15 minutes

2 tablespoons olive oil

½ cup chopped onion

6 ripe plum tomatoes, each cut into 6 slices

1 teaspoon sugar

½ teaspoon salt

1. Combine the rice beans with 4 cups water in a medium saucepan. Bring to a boil. Reduce the heat and simmer, partially covered, about 1½ hours or until tender, adding additional water if necessary. Drain.

2. Preheat the oven to the warm setting.

3. To cook the escarole, place it in a collapsible steamer basket set over simmering water in a wide saucepan. Cover and steam 5 to 8 minutes until tender. Drain and combine with the beans and salt in a serving bowl. Cover with foil and place in the oven to keep warm.

4. To prepare the sauce, drain the sun-dried tomatoes. Reserve the soaking liquid and cut the tomatoes in half.

5. Heat the oil in a medium nonstick skillet over medium heat. Add the onion and cook about 3 minutes, until tender. Add the fresh tomatoes and cook 5 minutes, stirring frequently. Stir in the sun-dried tomatoes, ¼ cup of the reserved liquid, the sugar, and salt. Cook 10 minutes longer.

6. Remove the escarole mixture from the oven and stir in the tomato mixture. Serve immediately.

SERVES 4

Kilocalories 331 Kc • Protein 17 Gm • Fat 8 Gm • Percent of calories from fat 21% • Cholesterol 0 mg • Dietary Fiber 6 Gm • Sodium 1108 mg • Calcium 192 mg

# White Beans with Escarole

*To serve as a main dish, toss with 1 pound cooked small pasta, such as shells or ditalini.*

1 bunch escarole (about 1½ pounds) trimmed and chopped

3 tablespoons extra-virgin olive oil

1 large garlic clove, minced

⅛ teaspoon red pepper flakes

3 cups cooked white beans

Salt

1. Cook the escarole in a large pot of boiling salted water for 5 minutes; drain well.

2. Heat the oil in a large skillet over low heat. Add the garlic and red pepper and cook until the garlic is just lightly browned, 2 to 3 minutes. Stir in the beans and escarole and cook about 3 minutes or until heated through. Season with salt to taste and serve immediately.

SERVES 4

**Kilocalories 306 Kc • Protein 15 Gm • Fat 11 Gm • Percent of calories from fat 31% • Cholesterol 0 mg • Dietary Fiber 14 Gm • Sodium 46 mg • Calcium 211 mg**

# Roasted Yams with Bok Choy and Beans

*I used pinto beans in this recipe, but use any bean you like, except chick-peas—they're too crunchy and strongly flavored for this dish. Our common sweet potato is often called a yam although technically it is not. Yams are a South American root vegetable which are hardly ever sold in this country. The name "yam" just seems so much more exotic than "sweet potato."*

1 large yam (about 1 pound), scrubbed, quartered length-wise, and cut into 1-inch slices
2 tablespoons dark sesame oil
2 teaspoons low-sodium soy sauce
¼ cup hoisin sauce
1 tablespoon minced fresh ginger

1 large garlic clove, minced
1 small head bok choy (about 1 pound), cut into ½-inch-thick slices
1 cup cooked beans, your choice
¼ cup finely chopped fresh cilantro

1. Preheat the oven to 500°.

2. Place the yam in an 11 × 7-inch baking pan coated with vegetable oil spray. Drizzle with 1 tablespoon of the sesame oil and toss to coat. Sprinkle with the soy sauce. Roast 10 to 15 minutes until tender and browned, stirring once.

3. Combine the hoisin sauce with ¼ cup water in a 1-cup measure. Set aside.

4. Heat the remaining 1 tablespoon oil in a large nonstick skillet or wok over medium-high heat. Add the ginger and garlic and cook 10 seconds. Add the bok choy and cook 5 minutes, stirring frequently. Pour the hoisin mixture over the bok choy, stir in the beans, and continue cooking until heated through, about 5 minutes. Turn off the heat and stir in the yams. Serve immediately.

SERVES 4

**Kilocalories 285 Kc • Protein 9 Gm • Fat 7 Gm • Percent of calories from fat 22% • Cholesterol 0 mg • Dietary Fiber 7 Gm • Sodium 141 mg • Calcium 175 mg**

# Sautéed Escarole and Cranberry Beans with Toasted Garlic Bread Crumbs

½ cup plain dried bread crumbs
¼ cup grated Romano cheese
2 tablespoons olive oil
2 garlic cloves, minced

1 bunch escarole, trimmed and
  coarsely chopped
2 cups cooked cranberry beans

1. Heat a large nonstick skillet over medium heat. Add the bread crumbs and stir constantly until lightly browned, about 3 minutes. Spoon the bread crumbs into a small bowl; add the cheese and stir to combine. Return the skillet to medium heat. Add the oil and garlic to the skillet; cook 1 minute until the garlic is just browned. Pour the mixture over the bread crumbs and cheese; stir to combine.

2. Return the skillet to medium heat; add the escarole, cover, and cook 5 minutes, stirring occasionally. Uncover, stir in the beans and cook until heated through, about 5 minutes. Sprinkle the bread crumb mixture over the escarole in the skillet; cover and cook 1 minute. Serve immediately.

SERVES 4

Kilocalories 276 Kc • Protein 13 Gm • Fat 10 Gm • Percent of calories from fat 31%
• Cholesterol 6 mg • Dietary Fiber 3 Gm • Sodium 219 mg • Calcium 179 mg

# Greens and Beans Burrito Casserole in Red Chili Sauce

*A delicious Tex-Mex dish. Serve with rice.*

*Sauce:*

1 tablespoon vegetable oil
1 large garlic clove, minced
⅓ cup chili powder
2½ cups reduced-sodium chicken
　or vegetable broth
2 tablespoons all-purpose flour
½ teaspoon salt

*Filling:*

1 tablespoon vegetable oil
¼ cup chopped onion
1 teaspoon cumin seeds
4 cups chopped green or red
　Swiss chard leaves
1½ cups cooked pinto, kidney, or
　black beans
1 cup cooked corn kernels
¼ cup chopped fresh cilantro

4 (8-inch) flour tortillas
1 cup reduced-fat shredded
　Cheddar cheese (about
　4 ounces)

1. Heat the oven to 375°.

2. To prepare the sauce, heat the oil in a medium nonstick skillet over medium heat. Add the garlic and cook 30 seconds. Add the chili powder, stirring constantly for 1 minute until a paste forms.

3. Gradually whisk the broth into the paste; cook (the sauce will boil), stirring occasionally, for 10 minutes. Whisk the flour together with ½ cup of the broth mixture until smooth. Stir into the skillet with the salt. Cook another 10 minutes until the mixture is reduced by half (about 1¼ cups).

4. To prepare the filling, heat the oil in a large skillet over medium heat. Add the onion and cumin seeds and cook about 30 seconds. Top with the Swiss chard, cover, and cook 3 to 5 minutes, stirring once, until the chard is wilted. Uncover, add the beans, corn, and cilantro. Remove from the heat and cool the mixture 10 minutes.

5. Spoon ¼ cup of the chili sauce into a 9-inch square baking dish. Fill each flour tortilla with equal amounts of the bean mixture (about 1 cup each) and sprinkle each with 2 tablespoons cheese; roll the tortilla around the filling and place seam side down in the baking dish. Pour the

remaining sauce over the tortillas and sprinkle with the remaining cheese; lightly cover with foil. Bake 10 minutes, remove the foil, and bake 10 minutes longer or until heated through.

SERVES 4

Kilocalories 467 Kc • Protein 23 Gm • Fat 17 Gm • Percent of calories from fat 32% • Cholesterol 20 mg • Dietary Fiber 8 Gm • Sodium 1475 mg • Calcium 472 mg

# Refried Greens and Beans

*Two cups of any steamed green may be substituted for the escarole in this recipe.*

1 tablespoons vegetable oil
½ cup chopped onion
3 cups cooked kidney or pinto beans
1 cup reduced-sodium vegetable broth
½ teaspoon freshly ground pepper

½ teaspoon salt
1 head escarole (about 1 pound), chopped and steamed
1 jalapeño pepper, seeded and finely chopped
½ cup shredded Cheddar cheese (about 2 ounces)

1. Heat the oil in a large nonstick skillet over medium heat. Add the onion and cook 1 to 2 minutes until tender.

2. Add 1½ cups of the beans and ½ cup of the broth to the skillet. Coarsely mash the beans with a potato masher. Add the remaining 1½ cups beans and ½ cup broth and mash. Stir in the pepper and salt. Cook, stirring frequently, about 5 minutes until the beans are thick. Reduce the heat to low; top with the greens and sprinkle with jalapeño peppers and cheese. Cover and cook 2 to 3 minutes until the cheese melts. Serve immediately.

SERVES 4

Kilocalories 289 Kc • Protein 18 Gm • Fat 8 Gm • Percent of calories from fat 25% • Cholesterol 15 mg • Dietary Fiber 4 Gm • Sodium 534 mg • Calcium 256 mg

# Steamed Broccoli Raab and Chickpea "Fries"

*Fries:*

2 cups cooked chickpeas
2 egg whites
1 tablespoon all-purpose flour
½ teaspoon ground cumin
½ teaspoon salt

¼ teaspoon freshly ground
   pepper

1 bunch broccoli raab, trimmed
   and chopped
Salt and freshly ground pepper

1. Combine all of the "fries" ingredients in a food processor fitted with the steel blade. Pulse until combined. Process 15 seconds until smooth. Spread evenly in an 8-inch baking pan coated with vegetable oil spray. Cut into eight 1-inch-wide rows then cut in half to form 16 "fries." Freeze 1 hour.

2. Preheat the oven to 500°.

3. Place the broccoli raab in a collapsible steamer basket set over simmering water in a wide saucepan. Cover and steam for 5 to 8 minutes. Turn the heat off but do not remove the steamer basket. Keep covered so that the broccoli raab will stay warm. Before serving, season with salt and pepper to taste.

4. Remove the chickpea mixture from the freezer. Run a sharp knife around the edge of the pan and cut through the edges of each slice to separate. Carefully unmold the chickpea mixture onto a baking sheet coated with vegetable oil spray. Use a flexible spatula underneath the frozen mixture to loosen any fries stuck to the pan. Coat the tops of the fries with additional spray. Bake for 15 minutes until browned. Serve immediately with the broccoli raab.

SERVES 4

Kilocalories 128 Kc • Protein 9 Gm • Fat 2 Gm • Percent of calories from fat 13%
• Cholesterol 0 mg • Dietary Fiber 7 Gm • Sodium 694 mg • Calcium 186 mg

# Roasted Red Peppers with Black-eyed Peas and Arugula in Warm Scallion Sauce

*I was fortunate enough to discover this wonderful recipe at the Lipstick Cafe in Manhattan. Chef Ron Gallo, a great guy, altered his recipe to fit this chapter and created two sauces to tantalize your taste buds.*

4 large red or yellow bell
  peppers
4 sprigs fresh thyme
4 garlic cloves, peeled
2 ears fresh corn in husks or
  1 cup cooked corn kernels
1 bunch arugula (about
  6 ounces), trimmed
1 cup cooked black-eyed peas
½ cup chopped red onion
½ cup chopped fresh cilantro
⅓ cup chopped fresh mint
1 bunch fresh chives, snipped
  (about ½ cup)

3 tablespoons champagne
  vinegar
1 tablespoon olive oil
¼ teaspoon salt
¼ teaspoon freshly ground
  pepper

*Warm Scallion Sauce:*

1 tablespoon salt
1 bunch scallions, trimmed
½ cup chicken or vegetable broth
2 tablespoons olive oil
Salt and freshly ground pepper

1. Preheat the oven to 400°.

2. Cut off the tops of the peppers; carefully remove the seeds and inner ribs, leaving the peppers whole. Place 1 sprig of thyme and 1 garlic clove in each pepper; place the peppers and corn in husks in a 13 × 9-inch roasting pan coated with vegetable oil spray. Roast about 40 minutes, turning every 10 minutes, until the peppers are lightly blistered and the corn is tender. Remove from the oven and wrap the pan tightly with foil. Let it stand 20 minutes.

3. Carefully peel the peppers, leaving them whole. Remove the thyme and garlic and discard. Shuck the corn and, with a sharp knife, cut the kernels from the cob. Place in a medium bowl.

4. Cut one fourth of the arugula into thin strips and add to the corn in the bowl. Stir in the peas, onion, cilantro, mint, chives, vinegar, oil, salt, and pepper. Spoon ½ cup of the mixture into each pepper. Divide the

remaining uncut arugula leaves among each pepper, stuffing the leaves inside with about 3 inches of the tops sticking out. Place each pepper on its side on a serving plate; spoon equal amounts of the remaining bean mixture onto the arugula.

5. To make the sauce, bring 2 inches of water plus 1 tablespoon salt to a boil in a wide saucepan; add the scallions and blanch 1 minute. Drain and run under cold water. Coarsely chop the scallions and place in a blender with the chicken broth, oil, salt, and pepper. Puree until smooth and creamy. Pour into a small saucepan and bring to a simmer over medium heat. Spoon ¼ cup sauce over each pepper and serve immediately.

SERVES 4

**Variation:** Warm Arugula-Walnut Sauce: 3 cups packed arugula leaves, 1 cup vegetable or chicken broth, 2 tablespoons grated Parmesan cheese, 2 tablespoons walnuts, 1 tablespoon olive oil, and 1 clove garlic. Place all of the ingredients in a blender and puree. Season with salt and freshly ground pepper to taste. Makes 2 cups (may also be used as a sauce for pasta).

Kilocalories 245 Kc • Protein 8 Gm • Fat 12 Gm • Percent of calories from fat 41% • Cholesterol 1 mg • Dietary Fiber 6 Gm • Sodium 185 mg • Calcium 150 mg

# 8

# International Greens

Worldwide, greens are vegetables that escape discrimination. They cross cultures and appear on the tables of every household, civilized and not so civilized. Wild greens, like mushrooms, have been foraged for centuries.

This chapter focuses on exotic ethnic cuisines that dress up and savor greens in unusual ways. From the rainforests of Brazil and the outback of Australia, to the woks of China and the street foods of Italy, to the stews of the Caribbean and the kettles of England and Ireland, greens are ubiquitous. Whether your preference is bok choy, arugula, cabbage, frisee, or dandelion, all have their special place in worldwide nutrition.

# Curried Spinach and Chickpeas

*There are different types of curry throughout the world, including Indian Madras, which is the hottest, and Jamaican, which is sweeter and more aromatic. As many as twenty spices, herbs, and seeds are crushed to make this special blend. Ethnic food shops carry the most authentic blends, but supermarket spices are a good substitute.*

1 tablespoon unsalted butter
2 cups coarsely chopped onion
2 tablespoons curry powder
1 package (10 ounces) frozen
    chopped spinach, thawed and
    drained

1 cup drained canned
    tomatoes with ½ cup
    juice
8 ounces cooked chickpeas
2 whole wheat chapati or
    pita breads

1. Melt the butter in a large saucepan over medium-high heat. Add the onion and cook 4 minutes, stirring frequently, until softened.

2. Stir in the curry powder and cook 1 minute. Add the spinach, tomatoes, and chickpeas with ½ cup water. Bring to a boil. Reduce the heat, cover, and simmer 10 minutes. Serve with the chapati.

SERVES 2

Kilocalories 502 Kc • Protein 21 Gm • Fat 11 Gm • Percent of calories from fat 19%
• Cholesterol 16 mg • Dietary Fiber 22 Gm • Sodium 1876 mg • Calcium 346 mg

# Colcannon

*I usually make colcannon the day after St. Patrick's Day. I often use left-over cooked potatoes and cabbage, which have been cooked with the corned beef, from the traditional holiday meal.*

2 pounds baking potatoes, pared
  and coarsely chopped
1 pound green cabbage,
  chopped
1 cup chopped leek (white part
  only)

1 cup skim milk
2 tablespoons unsalted butter
¾ teaspoon salt

1. Combine the potatoes, cabbage, and leek with 8 cups water in a large saucepan. Bring to a boil; reduce the heat to medium. Cook, partially covered, about 20 minutes until the potatoes are tender.

2. Drain the mixture and return to the pot. Add the milk, butter, and salt and mash together with a potato masher until creamy. Serve immediately.

SERVES 4

Kilocalories 320 Kc • Protein 9 Gm • Fat 7 Gm • Percent of calories from fat 18% • Cholesterol 17 mg • Dietary Fiber 5 Gm • Sodium 515 mg • Calcium 183 mg

# Chinese Stir-Fried Chicken and Flowering Kale

*Flowering kale is lovely with its bright lavender leaves edged in green. The kale adds a bit of crunch to this dish. If you don't have a wok, a large skillet will do.*

4 boneless chicken thighs (about 1 pound), cut into 1-inch strips
2 tablespoons cornstarch
½ teaspoon salt
2 tablespoons peanut oil
2 teaspoons minced fresh ginger

1 large garlic clove, minced
8 cups packed chopped flowering kale
2 tablespoons reduced-sodium soy sauce
Cooked brown rice, optional

1. Place the chicken on a length of wax paper. Sift the cornstarch and salt onto the chicken turning the pieces to coat; set aside.

2. Heat the oil in the wok over high heat. Add the chicken and cook 3 minutes, turning and separating the pieces. Add the ginger and garlic and cook 2 minutes, stirring frequently, until the chicken is no longer pink. Add the kale and soy sauce. Cook 3 minutes, stirring frequently. Serve with brown rice, if desired.

SERVES 4

Kilocalories 420 Kc • Protein 33 Gm • Fat 25 Gm • Percent of calories from fat 55% • Cholesterol 106 mg • Dietary Fiber 6 Gm • Sodium 729 mg • Calcium 139 mg

# Chinese Tofu, Lettuce, and Peanut Sauce

*This recipe also works well with shredded cooked chicken.*

*Peanut Sauce:*

½ cup creamy peanut butter
⅓ cup low-sodium chicken broth
2 tablespoons low-sodium soy
   sauce
2 tablespoons dry sherry
1 tablespoon rice wine
   vinegar
1 tablespoon sugar
1 tablespoon toasted sesame
   seeds

2 teaspoons minced fresh ginger
2 garlic cloves, minced
¼ teaspoon ground red pepper

*Salad:*

6 cups shredded iceberg lettuce
1 tablespoon dark sesame oil
2 cups cubed, drained firm tofu
½ cup sliced scallions (green and
   white), for garnish

1. Combine all of the sauce ingredients in a 2-cup measure.
2. Place the lettuce on a serving plate and drizzle with the sesame oil. Top with the tofu and drizzle with the peanut sauce. Garnish with the scallions and serve.

SERVES 4

Kilocalories 361 Kc • Protein 21 Gm • Fat 24 Gm • Percent of calories from fat 56% • Cholesterol 0 mg • Dietary Fiber 4 Gm • Sodium 556 mg • Calcium 111 mg

# Kale, Tofu, and Eggplant Stir-Fry

*Asian stir-fries, cooked in woks over high heat, rely on peanut oil because it has a higher smoke point.*

½ cup chicken broth
2 tablespoons hoisin sauce
1 pound tofu, drained and cubed
1 tablespoon peanut oil
½ teaspoon chili paste with garlic

2 cups diced eggplant
4 cups (packed) chopped kale
1 tablespoon chopped peanuts,
  optional

1. Combine the broth and hoisin sauce in a medium bowl. Add the tofu and let the mixture stand 15 minutes.

2. Heat the wok over high heat. Add the oil and swirl around until it starts smoking. Add the chili paste and cook 10 seconds. Add the eggplant and cook 3 minutes, until browned, stirring frequently. Add the kale and cook 2 minutes longer, stirring constantly.

3. Carefully add the tofu mixture and cook 5 minutes, stirring frequently. Top with the peanuts, if desired, and serve immediately.

SERVES 2

Kilocalories 305 Kc • Protein 23 Gm • Fat 13 Gm • Percent of calories from fat 38% • Cholesterol 1 mg • Dietary Fiber 8 Gm • Sodium 226 mg • Calcium 214 mg

# Stuffed Island Snapper

*Get a fabulous taste of the tropics in this Caribbean dish.*

1 (4-pound) dressed whole red snapper
1 teaspoon salt
½ teaspoon freshly ground pepper
¼ teaspoon ground allspice
¼ teaspoon ground cumin
¼ teaspoon ground ginger
1 cup freshly cooked white rice
1 cup cooked chopped kale
5 ounces frozen (thawed) whole baby shrimp
¼ cup sliced scallions
¼ cup shredded coconut
2 tablespoons chopped fresh cilantro
2 teaspoons grated fresh ginger
Scallion strips and cilantro leaves for garnish, optional
1 tablespoon vegetable oil

1. Preheat the oven to 350°.

2. Rinse the fish and pat it dry with paper towels. Combine the salt, pepper, allspice, cumin, and ginger in a small bowl. Rub the fish inside and out with the mixture.

3. Coat a 13 × 9-inch baking pan with vegetable oil spray. Place the fish in the pan.

4. Combine the rice, kale, shrimp, scallions, coconut, cilantro, and ginger in a medium bowl. Spoon the mixture into the cavity of the fish; place scallion strips and cilantro leaves on the fish, if desired. Tie the fish with twine and drizzle with the oil. Spoon any extra stuffing into the pan with the fish. Bake, uncovered, 30 to 35 minutes, until the fish is opaque. With a large, wide spatula, place the fish on a serving platter. Remove the twine and garnish with additional cilantro leaves, if desired.

SERVES 8

Kilocalories 363 Kc • Protein 64 Gm • Fat 7 Gm • Percent of calories from fat 17% • Cholesterol 107 mg • Dietary Fiber 1 Gm • Sodium 548 mg • Calcium 121 mg

# Asian Eggplant Stir-Fry

1 tablespoon vegetable oil
1 medium eggplant (about 1 pound), peeled and cut into ¾-inch cubes
1 cup shredded bok choy
1 tablespoon minced fresh ginger
1 large garlic clove, minced
½ cup chicken broth

1 tablespoon reduced-sodium soy sauce
½ teaspoon chili paste with garlic
12 ounces cubed cooked turkey breast or drained firm tofu
1 medium green bell pepper, cut into 1-inch pieces
½ teaspoon salt

1. Heat the oil in a wok or large skillet over high heat. Add the eggplant, bok choy, ginger, and garlic. Cook, stirring, for 1 minute.

2. Add the chicken broth, soy sauce, chili paste, turkey, and bell pepper to the wok. Reduce the heat to medium and cook 6 to 8 minutes, stirring often, until the pepper is tender. Stir in the salt and serve immediately.

SERVES 4

Kilocalories 200 Kc • Protein 29 Gm • Fat 5 Gm • Percent of calories from fat 21%
• Cholesterol 71 mg • Dietary Fiber 4 Gm • Sodium 513 mg • Calcium 59 mg

# Choucroute Garnie

Choucroute garnie *is a famous Alsatian sauerkraut dish usually served with a variety of pork products and potatoes, cooked in white wine. This recipe is definitely a variation on a theme. For a heartier meal, add cooked chicken sausage and chunks of cooked potatoes.*

1 cup thinly sliced onion
1 small Red Delicious apple, cored and cut into thin wedges
¾ cup mixed vegetable juice (6-ounce can)

1 tablespoon crushed fennel seeds
4 cups drained sauerkraut
8 turkey or meatless frankfurters, cut in half on the diagonal

1. Preheat the broiler.

2. Combine the onion, apple, vegetable juice, and fennel seeds in a large skillet. Cover and cook over medium-high heat until tender, 6 to 8 minutes, stirring occasionally. Reduce the heat and stir in the sauerkraut. Cook 3 minutes longer until heated through.

3. Place the franks on a rack in a pan. Broil 4 inches from the heat for 5 minutes, or until browned, turning once. Add to the skillet and serve immediately.

SERVES 4

Kilocalories 259 Kc • Protein 13 Gm • Fat 15 Gm • Percent of calories from fat 54% • Cholesterol 90 mg • Dietary Fiber 6 Gm • Sodium 2203 mg • Calcium 122 mg

# Malaysian Bobotie

*This dish is usually served with rice and chutney, but during the summer months a refreshing tropical fruit salad would be ideal.*

1 tablespoon peanut oil
1 medium summer squash, trimmed and diced (about 2 cups)
½ cup chopped onion
2 tablespoons Madras curry powder
1 teaspoon ground turmeric
¾ teaspoon salt
¼ teaspoon freshly ground pepper
1¼ pounds lean ground turkey

¼ cup chutney or apricot jam
3 tablespoons apple cider vinegar
2 slices whole wheat bread, cubed
¼ cup raisins
3 cups (packed) chopped fresh mustard greens
1 tablespoon chopped almonds
1 cup skim milk
1 large egg
4 bay leaves

1. Preheat the oven to 375°.

2. Heat the oil in a large nonstick skillet over medium heat. Add the squash and onion and cook 5 minutes, stirring frequently. Add the curry, turmeric, salt, and pepper and cook 1 minute.

3. Stir the turkey into the skillet and cook 5 minutes, breaking it up into little pieces with a wooden spoon. Add the chutney and vinegar, stirring until combined. Stir in the bread, then the raisins and top with the greens. Cover and cook 5 minutes, stirring occasionally. Uncover and stir in the almonds. Remove from the heat and spoon the mixture into a 2-quart casserole coated with vegetable oil spray.

4. Whisk the milk and egg together in a 1-cup measure; pour over the turkey mixture. Tuck in the bay leaves. Bake about 1 hour until browned and set. Let the dish stand 5 minutes before serving. Discard the bay leaves.

SERVES 4

Kilocalories 561 Kc • Protein 47 Gm • Fat 26 Gm • Percent of calories from fat 41% • Cholesterol 198 mg • Dietary Fiber 5 Gm • Sodium 732 mg • Calcium 218 mg

# Thai Chicken and Bok Choy in Coconut Milk

*Coconut milk is the unsweetened juice of the coconut meat. If the reduced-fat version is unavailable, dilute 1 cup of regular coconut milk with ½ cup of water. If you like your Thai food spicy, add another ¼ teaspoon red pepper flakes.*

2 teaspoons peanut oil
¼ teaspoon red pepper flakes
12 ounces chicken tenders, cut crosswise in half

1 bunch bok choy (about 1½ pounds), trimmed and chopped
1 can (14 ounces) reduced-fat coconut milk
½ teaspoon salt
4 cups cooked rice

1. Heat the oil in a large skillet or wok over medium-high heat. Add the red pepper flakes and cook 20 seconds until sizzling. Add the chicken and brown on all sides, about 2 minutes.

2. Stir in the bok choy and coconut milk. Reduce the heat, cover tightly, and simmer 15 minutes. Stir in the salt and serve immediately over the rice.

SERVES 4

Kilocalories 487 Kc • Protein 17 Gm • Fat 16 Gm • Percent of calories from fat 31% • Cholesterol 23 mg • Dietary Fiber 3 Gm • Sodium 839 mg • Calcium 246 mg

# Mahimahi with Bok Choy and Sweet and Sour Sauce

*Mahimahi hails from the shores of our 50th State, Hawaii. Although it's generally available, other firm-fleshed fish, such as halibut or grouper, may be substituted.*

4 mahimahi fillets, 1-inch thick
   (about 5 ounces each)
1 tablespoon fresh lemon juice
½ cup fresh orange juice
¼ cup chicken broth
2 tablespoons granulated sugar

1 tablespoon white wine vinegar
½ teaspoon dry mustard
1 tablespoon cornstarch
½ cup mandarin orange segments
1 head bok choy (about 1 pound),
   shredded and steamed

1. Preheat the broiler.

2. Place the fish on a rack in a pan, skin side down. Sprinkle with lemon juice. Broil 4 inches from the heat for 8 to 10 minutes, until the fish is opaque and tender.

3. To prepare the sauce, combine the orange juice, broth, sugar, vinegar, and mustard in a small saucepan and bring to a boil. Combine the cornstarch with 2 tablespoons of cold water in a small bowl and add to the hot mixture. Return to a boil over medium heat, stirring constantly; cook 1 minute. Remove from the heat and stir in the orange segments. Spoon the bok choy onto each of 4 serving plates. Top with the fish and drizzle with the sauce. Serve immediately.

SERVES 4

Kilocalories 224 Kc • Protein 35 Gm • Fat 2 Gm • Percent of calories from fat 7% • Cholesterol 62 mg • Dietary Fiber 1 Gm • Sodium 88 mg • Calcium 119 mg

# Mediterranean Swordfish with Arugula-Tomato Sauce (Outdoor Grill)

*This is topped with a raw tomato sauce which is known as* salsa cruda *in Italy.*

4 ripe medium tomatoes, diced
3 cups finely chopped arugula
8 kalamata olives, pitted and
chopped
2 tablespoons slivered fresh basil
1 tablespoon extra-virgin olive oil
1 tablespoon balsamic vinegar

1 large garlic clove, crushed
½ teaspoon salt
¼ teaspoon freshly ground
pepper
4 swordfish steaks, about ¾ inch
thick (5 ounces each)

1. Combine all of the ingredients except the swordfish in a medium bowl. Let the mixture stand at room temperature 1 hour.

2. Place the grill rack 5 inches from the coals and coat with vegetable oil spray. Prepare the grill, following the manufacturer's instructions. Grill the fish 3 to 4 minutes on each side or until it is done to your liking. Serve with the tomato sauce.

SERVES 4

Kilocalories 247 Kc • Protein 30 Gm • Fat 11 Gm • Percent of calories from fat 39% • Cholesterol 56 mg • Dietary Fiber 1 Gm • Sodium 511 mg • Calcium 49 mg

# Mexican Turkey Fajitas

*Fajitas are usually made with marinated steak. This recipe adapts deliciously to leftover turkey. The addition of tango lettuce, a very curly leaf variety, softens the bite of the picante sauce.*

8 ounces cooked turkey breast, cut in strips
3 tablespoons lime juice
1 large garlic clove, minced
½ teaspoon ground cumin
1 small onion, sliced
1 medium green bell pepper, cut into thin strips
2 teaspoons vegetable oil

¼ teaspoon salt
4 (8-inch) flour tortillas
1 cup chopped tango or leaf lettuce
1 cup coarsely shredded Monterey Jack cheese (about 4 ounces)
⅓ cup hot salsa

1. Combine the turkey strips, lime juice, garlic, and cumin. Let the mixture stand, covered, 1 hour.

2. Combine the onion, bell pepper, oil, and salt in a medium nonstick skillet coated with vegetable oil spray. Cook over medium heat for 10 to 15 minutes, until tender. Add the turkey to the skillet and cook until heated through, about 3 minutes.

3. Meanwhile, warm the tortillas in a toaster oven set at 200° for 3 minutes.

4. Spoon equal amounts of the turkey mixture onto each tortilla. Top each with equal portions of the greens, cheese, and salsa. Fold each tortilla over the filling and serve.

SERVES 4

Kilocalories 345 Kc • Protein 28 Gm • Fat 14 Gm • Percent of calories from fat 37% • Cholesterol 72 mg • Dietary Fiber 3 Gm • Sodium 651 mg • Calcium 287 mg

# Middle Eastern Stuffed Grape Leaves

*If you're lucky enough to find fresh grape leaves (I had a grapevine growing in my yard when I lived in Brooklyn), use them instead of the bottled variety. Choose tender, medium-size leaves. Trim, if necessary, and blanch in salted boiling water 2 to 3 minutes, until wilted. Rinse in cold water and drain thoroughly on paper towels.*

24 jarred grape leaves
10 ounces ground lean turkey
¼ cup finely chopped onion
2 heaping tablespoons long-grain
  rice (about 1 ounce)
2 tablespoons ketchup

1 tablespoon snipped fresh dill
2 teaspoons chopped pignoli nuts
1 teaspoon dried mint leaves
½ teaspoon minced garlic
1 tablespoon fresh lemon juice
Crumbled feta cheese, optional

1. Rinse the grape leaves and drain. Cut off the stems and discard. Place the leaves, vein side up, on paper towels.

2. Combine the turkey, onion, rice, ketchup, dill, pine nuts, mint, and garlic in a medium bowl. Place about 2 teaspoonfuls of the filling on each leaf, 1 inch from the stem end. Fold the stem end of the leaf over the filling, then fold the sides of the leaf over the filling and roll up jelly-roll fashion. Place, seam side down, in a Dutch oven.

3. Pour 2 cups of water over the leaves and sprinkle with the lemon juice. Bring to a boil. Reduce the heat and simmer, partially covered, for 45 minutes. Remove one roll and test for doneness (rice should be tender and turkey cooked through). Cool, cover, and refrigerate in the cooking liquid up to 3 hours. To serve, remove the rolls from the liquid and drain on paper towels. Garnish with cheese, if desired.

SERVES 6

Kilocalories 32 Kc • Protein 2 Gm • Fat 1 Gm • Percent of calories from fat 36%
• Cholesterol 5 mg • Dietary Fiber 0 Gm • Sodium 40 mg • Calcium 26 mg

# Greek Chicken En Papillote

*Food baked inside a wrapper, which is classically made of parchment paper, is referred to as "en papillote." If your kitchen isn't stocked with parchment, aluminum foil will work as well but won't look as dramatic on the plate as the puffed packet.*

6 cups chopped spinach
⅓ cup crumbled feta cheese
2 tablespoons chopped sun-dried
  tomatoes
1 tablespoon chopped pitted
  kalamata olives
1 large garlic clove, minced

4 boneless, skinless chicken
  breast halves (about 1¼
  pounds)
1 tablespoon fresh lemon
  juice
4 (12-inch) squares parchment
  paper
¼ teaspoon salt

1. Preheat the oven to 400°.

2. Add the spinach to a pot of boiling salted water. Cook 3 minutes. Drain, squeeze, and finely chop. Combine 2 tablespoons of the spinach with the cheese, tomatoes, olives, and garlic in a small bowl. Set aside.

3. Flatten each chicken breast to a ¼-inch thickness between wax paper. Spoon one fourth of the spinach-cheese mixture on one side of each chicken breast half. Fold the chicken over the filling and sprinkle with lemon juice.

4. Cut each piece of parchment paper into a 12-inch circle and coat with vegetable oil spray. Spoon one fourth of the remaining cooked spinach onto half of each circle and sprinkle with salt. Place one stuffed chicken breast on each mound of spinach. Fold the other half of the paper circle over the chicken. Seal the edges by turning them up and folding them together. Twist the ends a few times to secure the packet.

5. Bake on a baking sheet about 15 minutes or until the paper puffs up and is lightly browned. Place each packet on a serving plate, slit it open, and peel back the paper. Serve immediately.

SERVES 4

Kilocalories 317 Kc • Protein 50 Gm • Fat 10 Gm • Percent of calories from fat 29% • Cholesterol 139 mg • Dietary Fiber 3 Gm • Sodium 605 mg • Calcium 213 mg

# Greek Spinach and Cheese Triangles (Spanikopita)

*Silvia Lehrer, friend, cookbook author, and food columnist, contributed the following recipe, which I adapted. This main dish is delicious with a fresh tomato and orzo salad drizzled with an oregano-flecked vinaigrette.*

1 package (10 ounces) frozen chopped spinach, thawed, drained, and squeezed
½ cup part-skim ricotta cheese
¼ cup crumbled feta cheese
1 large egg

2 tablespoons finely chopped fresh dill (2 teaspoons dried)
¼ teaspoon salt
¼ teaspoon freshly ground pepper
6 sheets phyllo dough

1. To prepare the filling, combine the spinach, cheeses, egg, dill, salt, and pepper in a medium bowl.

2. Preheat the oven to 375°. Coat a baking sheet with vegetable oil spray.

3. Unroll the phyllo on a clean, dry counter with the short edge toward you. Cut lengthwise into thirds, each 4 inches wide; stack the strips into one pile. Coat the top strip with vegetable oil cooking spray. Place a tablespoon of the spinach filling at the bottom of each strip. Fold one corner of the strip over the filling diagonally to form a triangle; continue folding the triangle up the strip as you would fold a flag. Place a triangle on the prepared baking sheet. Lightly coat the top with cooking spray. Repeat with the remaining strips. Bake 15 to 18 minutes until browned and crisp. Serve immediately.

SERVES 3

Kilocalories 275 Kc • Protein 15 Gm • Fat 12 Gm • Percent of calories from fat 38% • Cholesterol 103 mg • Dietary Fiber 3 Gm • Sodium 766 mg • Calcium 356 mg

# Callaloo

*Callaloo is a popular Caribbean dish.*

2 cups low-sodium chicken broth
2 cups coarsely chopped fresh
  spinach
1 cup fresh or frozen corn kernels
1 cup sliced fresh okra (about 4
  ounces)
½ cup chopped onion

1 garlic clove, crushed
1 teaspoon fresh thyme
  (¼ teaspoon dried)
⅛ teaspoon Tabasco sauce
6 ounces fresh crabmeat
Salt and freshly ground pepper

Combine the broth, spinach, corn, okra, onion, garlic, thyme, and Tabasco with 2 cups water in a large saucepan. Bring to a boil; reduce the heat and simmer for 45 minutes. Add the crabmeat and simmer 15 minutes longer, stirring occasionally. Season with salt and pepper to taste and serve immediately.

SERVES 2

Kilocalories 225 Kc • Protein 24 Gm • Fat 4Gm • Percent of calories from fat 14% • Cholesterol 40 mg • Dietary Fiber 5 Gm • Sodium 858 mg • Calcium 152 mg

# German Cabbage and Chicken Stew

2 teaspoons vegetable oil
4 whole chicken legs (with thighs), skinned
1 cup sliced carrots
1 cup chopped onion
8 cups shredded savoy cabbage (1 small head)

1 tablespoon crushed caraway seeds, optional
Salt and freshly ground pepper
2 cups dark beer or chicken broth
1 tablespoon grainy mustard

1. Heat the oil in a large Dutch oven over medium heat. Add the chicken and cook 5 minutes, turning once to brown both sides. Remove the chicken to a plate.

2. Add the carrot and onion and cook 2 minutes, scraping the browned bits from the bottom of the pan. Stir in the cabbage, caraway seeds, salt, and pepper.

3. Whisk the beer and mustard together in a 4-cup measure and add it to the pot. Place the chicken on top. Turn the heat to high. When the mixture comes to a boil, reduce the heat and simmer, covered, for 45 minutes.

SERVES 4

Kilocalories 424 Kc • Protein 34 Gm • Fat 19 Gm • Percent of calories from fat 40%
• Cholesterol 105 mg • Dietary Fiber 7 Gm • Sodium 204 mg • Calcium 94 mg

# Steamed Bok Choy and Sesame Chicken

*Straw steamer baskets are sold in Asian markets and specialty stores. Two collapsible steamer baskets set in saucepans may be substituted.*

2 tablespoons dark sesame oil
2 garlic cloves, minced
1 tablespoon slivered fresh
  ginger
¼ teaspoon chili paste with garlic
1¼ pounds boneless, skinless
  chicken breasts, cut into
  1-inch cubes

1 head bok choy
  (about 1 pound)
1 bunch fresh cilantro or flat-leaf
  parsley
2 cups trimmed snow
  peas (about 6 ounces)
1 tablespoon reduced-sodium
  soy sauce

1. Combine the oil, garlic, ginger, and chili paste in a medium bowl; add the chicken to the mixture and toss to coat.

2. Line the bottom of two steamer baskets with the outer leaves of the bok choy. Chop enough of the remaining bok choy to make 2 cups; set it aside.

3. Place the chicken in one basket. Top with a second basket and fill it with the cilantro, chopped bok choy, and snow peas; cover. Lower the stack into a large wok or Dutch oven filled with 1 inch of boiling water (the water should not touch the food). Cover the wok and steam for 15 minutes or until the chicken is cooked. Remove the baskets from the water. With a slotted spoon, place the vegetables on each of 4 serving plates; top with the chicken and drizzle with the soy sauce. Serve immediately.

SERVES 4

Kilocalories 392 Kc • Protein 47 Gm • Fat 18 Gm • Percent of calories from fat 43%
• Cholesterol 119 mg • Dietary Fiber 3 Gm • Sodium 278 mg • Calcium 150 mg

# Chicken-Spinach Crepes With Mango Sauce

*Crepes:*

1 cup all-purpose flour
1 cup 1% milk
2 large eggs
1 tablespoon unsalted butter, melted
½ teaspoon salt

*Mango Sauce:*

2 medium mangoes, peeled and pitted
¾ cup vegetable or chicken broth
½ cup evaporated skimmed milk

2 teaspoons grated fresh ginger
¼ teaspoon salt

*Filling:*

3 cups cooked chicken, shredded
½ cup low-fat plain yogurt
½ (10-ounce) package frozen chopped spinach, thawed, drained, and squeezed
¼ cup grated fresh coconut or 2 tablespoons sweetened

1. Preheat the oven to the warm setting.

2. Whisk the flour, milk, eggs, butter, and salt together in a medium bowl.

3. Coat a crepe pan or an 8-inch nonstick sauté pan with vegetable oil spray. Heat the pan over medium-high heat until a drop of water sprinkled in the pan sizzles. For each crepe, pour a scant ¼ cup batter into the center of the pan, spreading with a spoon until a thin film covers the bottom. Cook 1 to 2 minutes or until the underside is light brown and dry. Run a spatula around the edges and lift the pancake out. Turn and cook about 30 seconds longer. Stack the pancakes on a plate as they are made and set aside.

4. Puree all of the sauce ingredients in a blender and set aside.

5. Combine all of the filling ingredients in a medium bowl. Mix well to combine. Fill each crepe with 3 tablespoons of the chicken mixture, roll up, and place in a 13 × 9-inch baking dish. Spoon the mango sauce over the top of the crepes and bake 15 to 20 minutes until heated through and bubbly.

SERVES 6

Kilocalories 353 Kc • Protein 31 Gm • Fat 10 Gm • Percent of calories from fat 25%
• Cholesterol 140 mg • Dietary Fiber 3 Gm • Sodium 569 mg • Calcium 196 mg

# Jamaican Crepes With Curried Greens Filling

*Crepes:*

1 cup skim milk
1 large egg
2 egg whites
¾ cup all-purpose flour
½ teaspoon baking powder
¼ teaspoon salt

*Filling:*

2 tablespoons vegetable oil

1 cup thinly sliced fresh mushrooms
½ teaspoon Jamaican curry powder
2 cups finely chopped greens (your choice)
12 ounces crumbled drained firm tofu
2 tablespoons reduced-sodium soy sauce
Chopped red bell pepper for garnish

1. Place all of the crepes ingredients in a blender (or whisk by hand). Process until smooth. Refrigerate 30 minutes.

2. Coat a crepe pan or an 8-inch nonstick skillet with vegetable oil spray. Heat over medium-high heat until a drop of water sizzles across the pan. For each crepe, pour ¼ cup of the batter into the center of the pan; immediately rotate the pan until the batter covers the bottom. Cook 1 to 2 minutes, until the underside is golden and dry; run a spatula around the edges and lift the pancake out. Turn and cook 1 minute longer. Cool on a rack. Repeat with the remaining batter, making 8 crepes. Stack the pancakes on a plate as they are made and set aside.

3. To prepare the filling, heat the oil in a medium skillet over medium-high heat. Add the mushrooms and curry; cook 5 minutes, stirring occasionally. Add the greens and cook 5 minutes longer, stirring frequently.

4. Combine the tofu and soy sauce in a small bowl. Add to the greens mixture and stir until it is heated through. Spoon equal amounts of filling onto each crepe. Fold or roll to enclose the filling.

Garnish with chopped bell pepper, if desired.

SERVES 4 (MAKES 8 CREPES)

Kilocalories 263 Kc • Protein 17 Gm • Fat 10 Gm • Percent of calories from fat 36% • Cholesterol 54 mg • Dietary Fiber 2 Gm • Sodium 633 mg • Calcium 186 mg

# Crepes With Salmon and Asian Mustard Greens

*Crepes:*

1 cup skim milk
1 large egg
2 egg whites
¾ cup all-purpose flour
½ teaspoon baking powder
¼ teaspoon salt

*Filling:*

8 ounces drained canned salmon (with bones)

1 cup finely chopped red Asian mustard greens or mizuna
2 tablespoons sliced scallions
2 tablespoons spicy brown mustard
1½ tablespoons soft tofu or light mayonnaise
¼ teaspoon salt
⅛ teaspoon freshly ground pepper

1. Place all of the crepes ingredients in a blender (or whisk by hand). Process until smooth. Refrigerate 30 minutes.

2. Coat a crepe pan or an 8-inch nonstick skillet with vegetable oil spray. Heat over medium-high heat until a drop of water sizzles across the pan. For each crepe, pour ¼ cup of the batter into the center of the pan; immediately rotate the pan until the batter covers the bottom. Cook 1 to 2 minutes, until the underside is golden and dry; run a spatula around the edges and lift the pancake out. Turn and cook 1 minute longer. Cool on a rack. Repeat with the remaining batter, making 8 crepes. Stack the pancakes as they are made on a plate and set aside.

3. To prepare the filling, combine the salmon, greens, and scallions in a medium bowl. Whisk the mustard, tofu, salt, and pepper in a small bowl; stir into the salmon mixture. Place about ¼ cup filling on each crepe. Fold or roll to enclose the filling.

SERVES 4 (MAKES 8 CREPES)

Kilocalories 253 Kc • Protein 21 Gm • Fat 8 Gm • Percent of calories from fat 30% • Cholesterol 92 mg • Dietary Fiber 2 Gm • Sodium 771 mg • Calcium 231 mg

# Italian Fish Stew

*This stew is popular in the seaport town of Livorno in northern Italy.*

1 tablespoon olive oil
½ cup sliced onion
3 garlic cloves, sliced
2 cups canned crushed
  tomatoes
¼ cup white wine vinegar
½ teaspoon salt
¼ teaspoon dried oregano
⅛ teaspoon ground red pepper
2 bay leaves

1 cup finely chopped dandelion
  greens
12 medium unshelled shrimp
12 littleneck clams, scrubbed
8 ounces halibut fillets, cut
  crosswise in 2-inch strips
8 ounces trimmed cleaned squid,
  cut crosswise in ½-inch strips
2 tablespoons coarsely chopped
  fresh flat-leaf parsley

1. Heat the oil in a Dutch oven over medium heat. Cook the onion and garlic about 3 minutes, until soft, stirring occasionally.

2. Add the tomatoes, vinegar, salt, oregano, pepper, bay leaves, and 1 cup water; reduce the heat and simmer 30 minutes, stirring frequently. During the last 15 minutes of cooking, add the dandelion greens.

3. Add the shrimp, clams, halibut, and squid and cook 5 minutes. Remove the bay leaves and garnish with the parsley. Serve immediately.

SERVES 4

Kilocalories 300 Kc • Protein 36 Gm • Fat 10 Gm • Percent of calories from fat 30%
• Cholesterol 180 mg • Dietary Fiber 3 Gm • Sodium 923 mg • Calcium 165 mg

# Baked Flounder Marinara

*In a pinch, one 10-ounce package of frozen greens, thawed and drained, may be substituted for the escarole.*

**4 flounder fillets (5 ounces each)**
**2 cups steamed escarole or dandelion greens**

**1½ cups drained canned stewed tomatoes, coarsely chopped**
**1 cup cooked peas**
**½ teaspoon dried oregano**

1. Preheat the oven to 400°.
2. Place the fish in an 8-inch square baking dish. Top with the escarole, tomatoes, and peas, spreading them evenly over the top. Sprinkle with the oregano. Bake, uncovered, for 12 to 15 minutes, or until the fish is opaque and tender.

SERVES 4

Kilocalories 266 Kc • Protein 34 Gm • Fat 8 Gm • Percent of calories from fat 26% • Cholesterol 86 mg • Dietary Fiber 4 Gm • Sodium 590 mg • Calcium 85 mg

# Polish Turkey Kielbasa With Sauerkraut

*Sauerkraut is the German word for "sour cabbage." To make sauerkraut from scratch is labor intensive. Cabbage and salt are placed in a stone crock and covered with cloth. It takes about a month to ferment, and the foam that rises to the top each day has to be removed. I recommend buying fresh sauerkraut at your local deli.*

| | |
|---|---|
| 1 (12-ounce) fully cooked turkey kielbasa | 2 cups thinly sliced onion |
| | 2 cups drained rinsed sauerkraut |
| 2 teaspoons vegetable oil | 2 teaspoons caraway seeds |

1. Preheat the oven to the warm setting.

2. Cut the kielbasa in half lengthwise, then in half crosswise to make 4 pieces. Brown for 2 to 3 minutes on each side over medium heat in a large nonstick skillet coated with vegetable oil spray. Place in an ovenproof casserole, cover with foil, and place in the oven.

3. Combine the oil and onion in the same skillet. Cook, covered, over low heat for 15 minutes, until soft. Uncover, turn the heat to medium and cook 3 to 5 minutes, stirring frequently, until browned. Add the sauerkraut and caraway seeds; cook 3 minutes longer or until heated through. Place the mixture around the kielbasa and serve. (The casserole may be covered and returned to the oven for up to 30 minutes before serving.)

SERVES 4

Kilocalories 186 Kc • Protein 15 Gm • Fat 9 Gm • Percent of calories from fat 45% • Cholesterol 53 mg • Dietary Fiber 4 Gm • Sodium 1181 mg • Calcium 23 mg

# Chinese Cabbage and Bamboo Shoots in Black Bean Sauce (Microwave)

*This recipe makes an easy and fast lunch or, if it is served over cooked rice or couscous, a light dinner.*

2 tablespoons fermented black bean sauce

2 cups shredded Chinese cabbage

1 can (8 ounces) sliced bamboo shoots, drained

4 ounces firm tofu, drained and cubed

1. Combine the black bean sauce with 1 tablespoon water in a small bowl.

2. Place the cabbage in a microwave-safe bowl; pour the black bean mixture over the cabbage. Cover with a lid or vented plastic wrap. Microwave on High for 3 minutes. Stir in the bamboo shoots and tofu and microwave on High for 2 minutes longer. Serve immediately.

SERVES 2

Kilocalories 92 Kc • Protein 9 Gm • Fat 3 Gm • Percent of calories from fat 29% • Cholesterol 0 mg • Dietary Fiber 4 Gm • Sodium 194 mg • Calcium 100 mg

# Cabbage and Chicken Scarpariello Style

*My friend Celia, a great cook, says that tongs are an indispensible piece of kitchen equipment. Since digging mine out of a box of infrequently used kitchen tools, I've discovered that she's right. They're much better than using a fork to turn small chicken pieces and to lift wilted greens from the pan.*

1 tablespoon vegetable oil
½ cup minced onion
3 garlic cloves, minced
1 3½ pound chicken, cut into about 30 pieces and skinned
½ teaspoon salt

½ teaspoon freshly ground pepper
1 cup distilled white vinegar
2 tablespoons chopped fresh rosemary (2 teaspoons dried)
4 cups shredded savoy cabbage

1. Heat the oil in a large nonstick skillet over medium heat. Add the onion and garlic and cook 1 minute until softened. Add the chicken and sprinkle with the salt and pepper. Brown 10 minutes on each side, turning with tongs.

2. Add the vinegar and rosemary, scraping the bottom of the pan to loosen any browned bits.

3. Reduce the heat and add the cabbage. Cover and simmer 10 minutes. Uncover, stir to combine, and cook 5 minutes longer.

SERVES 4

Kilocalories 785 Kc • Protein 110 Gm • Fat 30 Gm • Percent of calories from fat 37% • Cholesterol 329 mg • Dietary Fiber 3 Gm • Sodium 593 mg • Calcium 102 mg

# 9
# Entertaining and Party Foods

For some people, entertaining can be a daunting, anxiety-provoking proposition. For others, it presents an exciting challenge. The word "entertain" usually evokes an image of *haute cuisine* served to a tableful of sophisticated guests who will critique your cooking while you're in the kitchen trying to get the next course together. We often forget that entertaining takes many forms. An informal gathering of friends on a Friday night after a long work week should require little work and involve fuss-free foods, like good pizza and some premium ice cream. It's what I call "no-sweat" entertaining.

A lavish Saturday night cocktail party, on the other hand, calls for fancier food—the hors d'oeuvre. Like antipasto, a variety of these finger foods served with a party-size green salad adds up to a light meal. As a grand finale offer your guests a choice of desserts and coffee. Since the main course is eliminated, you can consider the desserts "freebies"—no calorie overload.

Finally, formal sit-down dinners tend toward more sophisticated preparations and presentation. You'll find many "wrapped up" meals in this chapter to suit the occasion. Wrapped food is full of expectation—the inside is a mystery waiting to unfold. Cutting into parchment, phyllo, or puff pastry yields steaming hot fillings and delights the diner with visual and sensual pleasure. Leafy greens also make wonderful wrappers. A salmon steak is no longer just a piece of fish when it's roasted in red chard.

In this chapter, you'll find a variety of food choices to match your personal entertaining style, calm your anxieties, and change your challenges into triumphs.

# Watercress-stuffed Mushrooms

*Often people ask if it's all right to wash mushrooms. The answer is yes. Some mushrooms have more soil on them than others and wiping them with a damp paper towel may not be enough. Rinse mushrooms (do not soak them) and be sure to dry them well before cooking.*

12 large fresh mushrooms
3 teaspoons olive oil
1 small shallot, minced
1 cup (packed) watercress leaves
2 teaspoons pignoli nuts
¼ teaspoon salt

2 tablespoons seasoned dried
  bread crumbs
1 tablespoon grated Romano
  cheese
1 tablespoon minced fresh flat-
  leaf parsley

1. Preheat the oven to 400°. Coat an 11 × 7-inch baking pan with vegetable oil spray.

2. Rinse and dry the mushrooms. Remove the stems and mince, setting the caps aside.

3. Heat 2 teaspoons of the oil in a medium nonstick skillet over medium heat. Add the minced mushroom stems and shallot and cook 5 minutes, stirring frequently. Add the watercress and cook 2 minutes longer, stirring occasionally. Stir in the nuts and salt, remove from the heat, and cool slightly.

4. Fill each mushroom cap with the watercress mixture and place in the prepared pan.

5. Combine the bread crumbs, cheese, and parsley on wax paper. Sprinkle onto the filled mushrooms. Drizzle with the remaining 1 teaspoon oil. Bake 20 to 25 minutes, until lightly browned. Serve warm.

SERVES 4

Kilocalories 69 Kc • Protein 2 Gm • Fat 5 Gm • Percent of calories from fat 62%
• Cholesterol 2 mg • Dietary Fiber 1 Gm • Sodium 56 mg • Calcium 37 mg

# Mozzarella-filled Radicchio Cups

*In this recipe I use fresh mozzarella, which is available in Italian specialty food markets. You may double the recipe for four servings.*

4 large radicchio leaves
3 ounces mozzarella, cut into
    ½-inch cubes
¼ teaspoon freshly ground
    pepper

⅛ teaspoon dried oregano
½ teaspoon crushed fennel
    seeds for garnish

1. Preheat the broiler. Coat an 11 × 7-inch baking pan with vegetable oil spray.

2. Fill the leaves with equal amounts of the cheese; sprinkle with the pepper and oregano. Coat each leaf with vegetable oil spray.

3. Place the pan on a broiler rack 4 inches from the heat. Broil 3 to 4 minutes, until the mozzarella begins to melt. Using a spatula, place on serving plates and sprinkle with the fennel seeds. Serve immediately.

SERVES 2

**Variation:** Let the stuffed cups cool to room temperature. Cut each cup in half and place on toasted Italian bread slices rubbed with cut garlic.

Kilocalories 124 Kc • Protein 9 Gm • Fat 9 Gm • Percent of calories from fat 67% • Cholesterol 33 mg • Dietary Fiber 0 Gm • Sodium 162 mg • Calcium 226 mg

# Spinach Dip in Pumpernickel

*My sister, Patti, makes a higher fat version of this dip for festive occasions. Everyone likes it so much that I was inspired to try a leaner interpretation. This recipe may be doubled.*

2 cups (16 ounces) plain nonfat yogurt

1 package (10 ounces) frozen leaf spinach, thawed, drained, and squeezed

1 cup low-fat or nonfat sour cream

2 tablespoons mayonnaise

4 scallions, trimmed and coarsely chopped

½ teaspoon salt

¼ teaspoon freshly ground pepper

⅛ teaspoon grated nutmeg

1 small round loaf pumpernickel bread

1. Place the yogurt in a sieve set over a bowl (a paper coffee filter also works well). Cover and refrigerate overnight.

2. Combine the strained yogurt with the remaining ingredients (except the bread) in a food processor. Process until smooth.

3. Cut off the top of the bread. Cut out the interior of the bread, leaving the outer crust. Cut the inner bread into 1-inch cubes. Fill the hollowed-out bread with the dip. Place on a large serving platter surrounded by the bread cubes.

SERVES 8

**Variation:** This dip is also a great low-fat sandwich spread. Spread the spinach mixture on 2 slices of Italian bread or a roll. Top with grilled vegetables or slices of ripe tomato in season.

Kilocalories 213 Kc • Protein 10 Gm • Fat 4 Gm • Percent of calories from fat 18% • Cholesterol 5 mg • Dietary Fiber 4 Gm • Sodium 553 mg • Calcium 236 mg

# Radicchio-filled Artichoke Bottoms

1 cup packed radicchio leaves
2 slices turkey or meatless salami
2 tablespoons snipped fresh
  chives or scallions
¼ teaspoon salt

1 tablespoon olive oil
2 cans (13¾ ounces each)
  artichoke bottoms, drained
10 radicchio leaves for
  garnish

1. Preheat the oven to 350°. Coat a 9-inch square baking pan with vegetable oil spray.

2. Mince the radicchio and turkey; combine with the chives and salt in a medium bowl.

3. Heat the oil in a medium skillet over medium heat. Add the radicchio mixture and cook 1 minute, stirring frequently.

4. Place the artichoke bottoms in the prepared pan and fill each with the mixture. Cover with foil and bake 15 minutes. Place each cup on a radicchio leaf and serve.

SERVES 4

Kilocalories 153 Kc • Protein 9 Gm • Fat 6 Gm • Percent of calories from fat 30%
• Cholesterol 12 mg • Dietary Fiber 10 Gm • Sodium 466 mg • Calcium 89 mg

# Sun-dried Tomato Cream Cheese and Belgian Endive

*Belgian endive is often confused with its closely related cousin, chicory. A native of India, it is grown in darkness to keep its creamy color from turning green.*

¼ cup sun-dried tomato bits
1 cup low-fat cream
   cheese
1 tablespoon minced fresh
   basil (1 teaspoon dried)

1 tablespoon dry sherry (or
   water)
16 endive leaves (about 2 large
   heads)
Fresh basil leaves for garnish

1. Combine the tomatoes and ¼ cup water in a small saucepan over medium heat. Bring to a boil. Remove from the heat and cool completely. Drain.

2. Combine the tomatoes, cream cheese, basil, and sherry in a small bowl.

3. Spread about a tablespoon of the mixture onto the base end of each endive. Place 4 endive leaves on each of 4 plates and garnish the plates with basil leaves.

SERVES 4

**Variation:** ½ cup nonfat cream cheese, ¼ cup creamy Gorgonzola cheese, 1 tablespoon minced fresh parsley, and ½ teaspoon freshly ground pepper. Combine all of the ingredients and spread on endive (24 leaves). This recipe is higher in fat, so spread a thin layer of the mixture onto each leaf. Serves 8.

**Variation 2:** ½ cup low-fat cream cheese, ¼ cup Indian mango chutney, 1 tablespoon minced fresh sorrel, and a pinch of ground red pepper. Combine all of the ingredients and spread on endive (12 leaves). Serves 6.

Kilocalories 162 Kc • Protein 7 Gm • Fat 10 Gm • Percent of calories from fat 59% • Cholesterol 30 mg • Dietary Fiber 2 Gm • Sodium 372 mg • Calcium 94 mg

# Macadamia Spinach and Belgian Endive

*Vegetable or olive oil is not a good substitute in this recipe. Macadamia nut oil lends a very special flavor to the dish. It can be found in health food and specialty food stores.*

3 teaspoons macadamia nut oil
¼ cup minced onion
3 tablespoons finely chopped
    macadamia nuts
1 package (10 ounces) frozen
    chopped spinach, thawed,
    drained, and squeezed

¼ teaspoon salt
1 tablespoon mayonnaise
16 endive leaves (about
    2 heads)
1 cup diced tomato
4 whole macadamia nuts

1. Heat 2 teaspoons of the oil in a medium nonstick skillet over medium heat. Add the onion and chopped nuts; cook 1 minute. Add the spinach and salt, stirring constantly to break up any clumps, and cook 2 minutes longer. Remove from the heat and cool.

2. Whisk the mayonnaise together with the remaining 1 teaspoon oil and 2 teaspoons of cold water in a 1-cup measure.

3. Arrange 4 endive leaves on each of 4 salad plates, in a circle, with the leaf bases touching in the center.

4. Shape the spinach mixture into 4 equal balls, pressing to keep them together. Place one in the center of each plate. Sprinkle ¼ cup tomato around each ball and drizzle the tomatoes with the mayonnaise dressing. Place one macadamia nut on top of each spinach ball. Serve at room temperature.

SERVES 4

Kilocalories 151 Kc • Protein 4 Gm • Fat 12 Gm • Percent of calories from fat 64%
• Cholesterol 3 mg • Dietary Fiber 5 Gm • Sodium 232 mg • Calcium 124 mg

# Watercress Cocktail Sandwiches

*These hors d'oeuvres may also be served as tea sandwiches.*

3 tablespoons whipped
   unsalted butter, at room
   temperature
½ teaspoon lemon
   pepper

6 thin slices whole wheat bread,
   crusts removed
½ cup (packed) chopped
   watercress
Watercress sprigs for garnish

1. Combine the butter and lemon pepper in a small bowl. Spread 2 teaspoons of the mixture on each slice of bread. Top 3 slices of the bread with equal amounts of watercress. Cover each with a top slice and press to close. Wrap each sandwich in plastic wrap and place in a sealable plastic bag. Refrigerate up to 24 hours.

2. To serve, bring the sandwiches (wrapped) to room temperature. Cut each sandwich on the diagonal into 4 slices to form triangles. Place the watercress sprigs in the center of a serving plate. Place the sandwiches around the rim of the plate. Serve immediately.

SERVES 4

Kilocalories 173 Kc • Protein 4 Gm • Fat 11 Gm • Percent of calories from fat 53%
• Cholesterol 25 mg • Dietary Fiber 3 Gm • Sodium 201 mg • Calcium 35 mg

# Watercress-Walnut Spread on Mini Bagels

*This spread is also good on bagel chips, jicama slices, or stuffed into celery.*

8 ounces low-fat cream cheese,
  at room temperature
1 cup finely chopped, trimmed
  watercress

¼ cup minced scallions
¼ cup chopped
  walnuts
12 mini bagels

1. Combine the cream cheese, watercress, scallions, and walnuts in a small bowl. Refrigerate the spread until ready to use. Let it stand at room temperature 1 hour before serving.

2. Slice the bagels and spread with the watercress cream cheese. Serve immediately.

SERVES 12 (1½ CUPS SPREAD)

**Variation:** Watercress Butter: Place ½ cup whipped unsalted butter, ½ cup (packed), trimmed watercress, and ¼ teaspoon salt in a mini food processor. Process until smooth. Cover and refrigerate. A small pat of this butter on grilled foods goes a long way.

Kilocalories 128 Kc • Protein 7 Gm • Fat 2 Gm • Percent of calories from fat 16%
• Cholesterol 1 mg • Dietary Fiber 1 Gm • Sodium 268 mg • Calcium 45 mg

# Mini Meatballs

*These meatballs are terrific with the Cherry Tomato Sauce on page 198. Although basically spinach, this meatball is mixed with turkey and uses rice as a binder instead of bread crumbs.*

1 tablespoon olive oil
1 garlic clove, minced
2 cups (packed) finely chopped spinach
8 ounces ground lean turkey
½ cup cooked brown or white rice
1 large egg

¼ cup grated Romano cheese
¼ cup chopped fresh flat-leaf parsley
¼ teaspoon salt
¼ teaspoon freshly ground pepper
2 cups cooked tomato sauce, preferably homemade

1. Heat the oil in a large nonstick skillet over medium heat. Add the garlic and cook 30 seconds until lightly browned. Stir in the spinach. Reduce the heat, cover, and cook until the spinach is wilted, about 5 minutes.

2. Combine the turkey, rice, egg, cheese, parsley, salt, and pepper in a medium bowl. Stir in the spinach. Form the mixture into thirty-two 1-inch meatballs.

3. Wipe out the skillet and spray with vegetable oil spray. Place over medium heat. Add the meatballs and cook about 10 minutes, turning gently to brown on all sides. Add the sauce, reduce the heat, cover, and simmer 5 minutes until hot and bubbly and the meatballs are cooked through. Serve immediately.

SERVES 8 (MAKES 32 MEATBALLS)

Kilocalories 117 Kc • Protein 8 Gm • Fat 6 Gm • Percent of calories from fat 44% • Cholesterol 52 mg • Dietary Fiber 1 Gm • Sodium 532 mg • Calcium 65 mg

# Mustard Greens and Swiss Cheese Balls (Microwave)

2 teaspoons vegetable oil
1 teaspoon crushed caraway
  seeds
1 small shallot, minced
1 package (10 ounces) chopped
  frozen mustard greens, thawed
½ cup (2½ ounces) shredded
  Swiss cheese
½ cup plain dried bread crumbs
2 large egg whites

¼ teaspoon salt
¼ teaspoon freshly ground
  pepper

*Dip:*

¾ cup applesauce
2 tablespoons vanilla
  yogurt

1. Heat the oil in a small skillet over medium heat. Add the caraway seeds and shallot and cook about 1 minute until the shallots are soft. Set aside.

2. Remove the paper from the package of greens. Microwave the package on High for 4 to 5 minutes or until defrosted. Cool and squeeze the greens of all liquid.

3. Mix the greens with the reserved caraway mixture, the cheese, bread crumbs, egg whites, salt, and pepper in a medium bowl. Shape into twenty-four 1-inch balls. Place in a single layer in a baking pan; cover and freeze overnight. (The balls may be frozen up to 2 weeks.)

4. To prepare the dip, combine the applesauce and yogurt in a small bowl. Microwave on High for 1 to 2 minutes, rotating once. Cover and keep warm.

5. To serve the cheese balls, place a paper towel on a microwave-safe dinner plate and top with the frozen balls. Microwave on High for 2 minutes. Reduce the power to Medium and microwave for 5 to 6 minutes, rotating the dish if necessary once or twice, until the balls are hot. Remove the paper towel and serve, with the dip, immediately or the balls will become rubbery.

SERVES 6

Kilocalories 125 Kc • Protein 7 Gm • Fat 5 Gm • Percent of calories from fat 38% • Cholesterol 11 mg • Dietary Fiber 2 Gm • Sodium 240 mg • Calcium 195 mg

# Mache and Crab Cocktail

*Mache is alternately known as corn salad and lamb's lettuce. It is slightly nutty in flavor and very tender.*

*Sauce:*

¾ cup part-skim ricotta cheese
1 tablespoon vegetable oil
1 tablespoon fresh lemon juice
2 teaspoons Worcestershire
   sauce
2 teaspoons Dijon mustard
2 teaspoons brandy, optional
⅛ teaspoon Tabasco sauce

*Cocktail:*

Bibb lettuce leaves
6 ounces cooked crabmeat
1 cup drained rinsed bean
   sprouts
½ cup coarsely chopped
   mache
1 tablespoon snipped fresh
   chives or scallions

1. Combine all of the sauce ingredients in a small food processor fitted with the steel blade. Process until smooth. Cover and refrigerate up to 4 hours.

2. To serve, line 4 salad plates with lettuce leaves. Spoon equal amounts of crab, sprouts, mache, and chives onto the lettuce. Spoon about ¼ cup sauce over each plate and serve.

SERVES 4

Kilocalories 141 Kc • Protein 14 Gm • Fat 8 Gm • Percent of calories from fat 48% • Cholesterol 33 mg • Dietary Fiber 1 Gm • Sodium 454 mg • Calcium 146 mg

# Samosas

*Samosas are potato-filled Indian turnovers that are usually deep-fried. These samosas, however, are baked in a dough made with almost no fat. The filling is traditional with the exception of the leafy greens. Although this recipe uses sorrel, which adds an unusual lemony, slightly sour taste, spinach would be an excellent substitute.*

*Dough:*

2 cups all-purpose flour
½ teaspoon salt
¾ cup low-fat buttermilk
1 teaspoon vegetable oil

*Filling:*

2 medium potatoes (about 6
  ounces each), pared and diced

3 tablespoons vegetable oil
½ cup finely chopped onion
2 tablespoons minced fresh
  ginger
1 teaspoon coriander seeds
6 cups chopped sorrel
½ cup cooked fresh peas or
  uncooked frozen peas
1 teaspoon salt

1. Combine the flour and salt in a food processor fitted with the steel blade. Pour in the buttermilk and oil and pulse until a ball forms. Process the dough 40 seconds to knead. Flatten the dough, wrap in plastic wrap, and refrigerate overnight. Remove the dough from the refrigerator 30 minutes before use.

2. To prepare the filling, place the potatoes in a collapsible steamer basket set over simmering water in a wide saucepan. Cover and steam 5 to 8 minutes, until tender. With a fork, carefully remove the basket from over the water and place in the sink.

3. Heat the oil in a large nonstick skillet over medium heat. Add the onion, ginger, and coriander and cook 3 minutes, stirring frequently. Turn the heat to medium-high and add the potatoes. Cook 5 minutes, stirring frequently, until lightly browned. Stir in the sorrel, peas, and salt. Cover and cook 5 minutes longer. Remove from the heat, uncover, stir the mixture, and let it cool completely.

4. Preheat the oven to 425°. Coat a baking sheet with vegetable oil spray and set aside.

5. Lightly flour a large surface and a rolling pin. Roll the dough, which will be slightly sticky, to a ¼-inch thickness; sprinkle with flour, lift and turn over onto a newly floured surface (to prevent sticking). Roll the dough to a ⅛-inch thickness. With a 4-inch cutter, cut circles. Roll each circle into a 5-inch round and place 1 heaping tablespoon of the sorrel mixture in the center and fold it over into a half-moon shape. Seal the edges with the tines of a fork. Place each turnover on the prepared pan. Coat each turnover with vegetable oil spray. Bake 15 minutes, reduce the heat to 375°, and bake 8 to 10 minutes longer until browned and crisp. Serve warm.

SERVES 6 (MAKES 18 SAMOSAS)

**Kilocalories 266 Kc • Protein 10 Gm • Fat 3 Gm • Percent of calories from fat 9% • Cholesterol 1 mg • Dietary Fiber 4 Gm • Sodium 625 mg • Calcium 95 mg**

# Green Olive Paste and Arugula on Toast

*Olive paste:*

30 large green Greek olives, pitted
3 tablespoons whole blanched almonds
1 tablespoon olive oil
1 medium garlic clove, mashed
1 tablespoon raisins

1 teaspoon fresh lemon juice
¼ teaspoon ground cumin
¼ teaspoon ground cloves

24 melba toast rounds or thin whole wheat toast, cut in quarters
½ cup minced arugula

1. Combine all of the olive paste ingredients in a food processor fitted with the steel blade. Process until almost smooth, scraping down the sides of the bowl.

2. Transfer the mixture to a bowl and pound with a pestle until the mixture forms a paste. Cover and refrigerate.

3. To serve, spread a thin layer of the olive paste on the rounds of bread. Mound each with the arugula and serve immediately.

SERVES 8 (MAKES 1¼ CUPS)

Kilocalories 121 Kc • Protein 3 Gm • Fat 6 Gm • Percent of calories from fat 43% • Cholesterol 0 mg • Dietary Fiber 1 Gm • Sodium 405 mg • Calcium 56 mg

# Sorrel and Tomato Mousse

*This two-tone, two-layer mousse is scrumptious. The best part is that all the work is done the day before you serve it. To serve, unmold it onto a large platter and surround the mousse with endive leaves and cucumber and carrot slices. For a fancier touch, unmold the mousse onto a footed pedestal dish, top with caviar, and serve with water crackers.*

10 ounces sorrel, stems removed
¼ cup vegetable broth
2 envelopes unflavored gelatin
   (or equivalent agar-agar)
3 tablespoons heavy cream
1 cup part-skim ricotta cheese
1 cup nonfat cream cheese
1½ tablespoons snipped fresh dill

1 tablespoon fresh lemon
   juice
Salt
Freshly ground pepper
2 ripe medium tomatoes, peeled,
   seeded, and pureed
Dill sprigs and diced tomato for
   garnish

1. Combine the sorrel and broth in a medium saucepan. Cover and bring to a boil. Remove from the heat and cool. Drain, reserving the liquid. Puree the sorrel in a blender or food processor. Dissolve the gelatin in the reserved broth and set it aside.

2. Whip the cream in a small bowl with an electric mixture until just stiff. Stir in the cheeses, dill, lemon juice, salt, pepper, and dissolved gelatin. (If the gelatin hardens, dissolve again over very low heat).

3. Place half of the cheese mixture (about a cup) in another bowl. Stir in the sorrel until blended. Add the tomato to the other half of the cheese mixture, stirring to combine.

4. Spoon the tomato mixture into the bottom of a 4-cup mold. Top with the sorrel mixture. Cover and refrigerate overnight. To unmold, run a knife around the rim of the pan. Place a plate on top of the mold, and holding both tightly, invert the plate and mold. Shake gently, then carefully remove the mold. Repeat the process, if necessary. Garnish with tomato and dill and serve.

SERVES 8

**Variation:** Finely chop 2 ounces of smoked salmon and stir into the tomato mousse mixture. This makes a great brunch dish.

**Kilocalories 99 Kc • Protein 10 Gm • Fat 4 Gm • Percent of calories from fat 35%**
**• Cholesterol 8 mg • Dietary Fiber 1 Gm • Sodium 192 mg • Calcium 172 mg**

# Spinach-Chickpea Spread

*This spread is made with yogurt cheese. It's delicious on whole wheat pita toasts.*

1 cup plain low-fat yogurt
1 cup coarsely chopped fresh spinach
½ cup drained cooked chickpeas

½ teaspoon salt
¼ teaspoon toasted mustard seeds
⅛ teaspoon freshly ground pepper

1. Line a sieve with paper towels; place over a medium bowl and add the yogurt (a paper-lined coffee filter works well, too). Cover and refrigerate overnight. Pour off and discard any liquid. Spoon the yogurt from the sieve into the bowl.

2. Combine the spinach and chickpeas in a food processor fitted with the steel blade. Process until the spinach is finely chopped and the mixture is smooth. Add the spinach mixture to the yogurt and stir in the salt, mustard seeds, and pepper. Serve at room temperature.

SERVES 3 (1¼ CUP SPREAD)

**Variation:** Make the yogurt cheese. Combine ½ cup drained canned water-packed tuna, ½ cup chopped fresh spinach, and 2 tablespoons chopped celery in a food processor. Process until finely chopped. Stir the spinach mixture and 1 tablespoon grainy mustard into the yogurt cheese. Add pepper to taste.

Kilocalories 76 Kc • Protein 6 Gm • Fat 1 Gm • Percent of calories from fat 9% • Cholesterol 1 mg • Dietary Fiber 2 Gm • Sodium 573 mg • Calcium 182 mg

# Savory Cottage Cheese Dip

*The perfect low-fat centerpiece for a platter of raw vegetables or a good filling for a pita pocket.*

½ cup whole trimmed radishes
½ cup coarsely chopped carrots
½ cup mache (or watercress)
¼ cup coarsely chopped scallions

2 cups low-fat cottage cheese
½ teaspoon chili powder

1. Place the radishes, carrots, mache, and scallions in a food processor fitted with the steel blade. Process until finely chopped. Add the cottage cheese and chili powder and process until creamy. Refrigerate, covered, until ready to serve.

2. To serve, let the dip stand at room temperature 1 hour.

SERVES 4 (1½ CUPS DIP)

Kilocalories 93 Kc • Protein 14 Gm • Fat 1 Gm • Percent of calories from fat 12% • Cholesterol 5 mg • Dietary Fiber 1 Gm • Sodium 471 mg • Calcium 84 mg

# Grilled Oysters with Spinach Pesto (Outdoor Grill)

*For a colorful presentation, spoon finely chopped roasted peppers or a little bit of diced tomato salad in the center of each plate. Arrange 6 oysters around the rim of the plate.*

**24 medium oysters**

*Spinach Pesto:*

**¼ cup (packed) chopped fresh spinach**
**1 tablespoon pignoli nuts**

**2 teaspoons grated Romano cheese**
**2 teaspoons olive oil**
**1 small garlic clove**
**⅛ teaspoon salt**
**⅛ teaspoon freshly ground pepper**

1. Place the grill rack 5 inches from the coals and coat with vegetable oil spray. Prepare the grill following the manufacturer's instructions.

2. Scrub the oyster shells under cold running water. Discard any oysters whose shells are not tightly closed. Place in a plastic bag and refrigerate until ready to use.

3. Puree all of the pesto ingredients in a small food processor and set aside.

4. Place the oysters on the grill rack, flat shell up, over the hot coals. Grill 4 to 6 minutes, or until the shells open slightly. Discard any oysters that do not open. Carefully remove the oysters with tongs, not spilling any juices. Place on a platter.

5. Wearing an oven mitt, hold each oyster flat side up and pull off the top shell. It may be necessary to loosen the top shell with a small knife. Spoon a scant ½ teaspoon of the pesto onto each oyster and serve.

SERVES 4

Kilocalories 97 Kc • Protein 7 Gm • Fat 6 Gm • Percent of calories from fat 54% • Cholesterol 45 mg • Dietary Fiber 0 Gm • Sodium 267 mg • Calcium 54 mg

# Mexican Mini Bagels

*Queso quesadilla is a tasty semi-soft cheese that is shreddable. Monterey Jack cheese is a good standby, if the Queso cheese is unavailable.*

10 mini bagels, sliced
¼ cup jalapeño jelly (or other hot and spicy jelly)
¾ cup steamed spinach, squeezed of excess liquid and finely chopped

Kosher or coarse salt
¾ cup shredded Queso quesadilla cheese (about 3 ounces)

1. Preheat the oven to 375°.
2. Spread each bagel half with a thin layer of jelly. Top each with a little spinach and sprinkle with a pinch of salt. Top with the cheese. These may be made up to 1 hour ahead. Place in a baking pan to fit. Bake 15 minutes. Let the bagels stand 5 minutes before serving.

SERVES 6

Kilocalories 250 Kc • Protein 10 Gm • Fat 5 Gm • Percent of calories from fat 18% • Cholesterol 13 mg • Dietary Fiber 2 Gm • Sodium 415 mg • Calcium 153 mg

# Stuffed Baguette Slices

*This is perfect party food. If you're having other hors d'oeuvres along with the baguettes, this can easily serve 10 to 12.*

*Red Pepper Mayonnaise:*

1 large garlic clove
¼ cup roasted red peppers
½ teaspoon balsamic vinegar
½ cup light mayonnaise
¼ teaspoon salt
¼ teaspoon freshly ground
    pepper

*Baguette Filling:*

3 cups thinly sliced fresh
    mushrooms (about 8
    ounces)
1 tablespoon balsamic vinegar
¼ teaspoon salt
1 thin French baguette (22 inches
    long and 2 inches wide)
1 cup finely chopped arugula
Additional arugula leaves for
    garnish, optional

1. To prepare the mayonnaise, mince the garlic in a small food processor. Add the peppers and vinegar and process until smooth. Add the mayonnaise, salt, and pepper and pulse until combined. Spoon the mixture into a small bowl and refrigerate, covered, until ready to use.

2. To prepare the filling, combine the mushrooms, vinegar, and salt with 2 tablespoons water in a medium nonstick skillet. Cover and cook over high heat for 3 to 5 minutes until the mushrooms are soft. Uncover, stir, and cook 2 minutes longer or until the liquid is absorbed.

3. Slice the baguette horizontally with a serrated knife. Remove the soft interior of the bread from the top and bottom, leaving the crusts to form a shell.

4. Spread both shells with equal amounts of the mayonnaise mixture. Fill the bottom shell with the mushrooms and arugula to within 2 inches of each end. Press the top shell onto the filled baguette. Wrap the baguette in foil and refrigerate at least 4 hours or overnight.

5. To serve, trim 2 inches from each end of the baguette and discard. Cut the baguette into 1-inch-thick slices with a serrated knife. Place a toothpick through each slice to hold it together, if necessary. Place the

slices on a serving platter around a small mound of arugula leaves and serve immediately.

SERVES 6 (ABOUT 20 SLICES)

**Kilocalories 207 Kc • Protein 6 Gm • Fat 8 Gm • Percent of calories from fat 34% • Cholesterol 0 mg • Dietary Fiber 1 Gm • Sodium 652 mg • Calcium 10 mg**

# Crostini With Cabbage and Olives

*This cabbage mixture is versatile. It is terrific tossed with pasta and olive oil, added to potato soup, or as a topping for grilled tofu.*

9 (½-inch-thick) slices Italian bread
1 large garlic clove, cut in half
   lengthwise
3 cups finely chopped cabbage
½ cup vegetable broth

10 pimiento-stuffed olives,
   chopped
1 teaspoon extra-virgin olive oil
¼ teaspoon kosher or
   coarse salt

1. Preheat the oven to 400°.
2. Place the bread on a baking sheet. Bake 12 to 15 minutes until lightly browned. Rub each slice with a cut side of the garlic.
3. Combine the cabbage and broth in a large nonstick skillet. Cover and cook over medium-low heat about 8 minutes, stirring occasionally, until the broth has evaporated and the cabbage is lightly browned. Remove from the heat and stir in the olives.
4. Top each bread slice with about 1 tablespoon of the cabbage mixture. Drizzle each with a little oil, sprinkle with salt, and serve.

SERVES 3

**Kilocalories 298 Kc • Protein 9 Gm • Fat 6 Gm • Percent of calories from fat 19% • Cholesterol 0 mg • Dietary Fiber 4 Gm • Sodium 873 mg • Calcium 118 mg**

# Crostini with White Beans and Dandelion

*Greens and beans are a staple of the cuisine of the southern regions of Italy, while crostini (little toasts) are found in the north. Combining these ingredients offers the best of both.*

8 (½-inch-thick) slices Italian bread
1 large garlic clove, sliced in half lengthwise
1 cup (packed) dandelion greens
½ cup cooked cannellini beans (if canned, rinse and drain)
2 teaspoons extra-virgin olive oil
1 tablespoon fresh lemon juice
¼ teaspoon salt
⅛ teaspoon freshly ground pepper

1. Preheat the oven to 400°.
2. Place the bread on a baking sheet. Bake 12 to 15 minutes until lightly browned. Rub each slice with a cut side of the garlic.
3. Place the dandelion greens in a collapsible steamer basket set over simmering water in a wide saucepan. Cover and steam 5 minutes until bright green. Carefully remove the steamer basket and place in the sink. Cool the greens slightly. Place in paper towels and gently squeeze to remove the excess liquid. Place the greens on a small cutting board and finely chop.
4. Mash the beans in a medium bowl. Stir in the dandelion greens, oil, lemon juice, salt, and pepper.
5. Spread the bean mixture evenly over the bread slices and serve.

SERVES 4

**Variation:** Crab and Radicchio: Follow steps 1 and 2. Combine 3 ounces cooked crabmeat, 2 tablespoons finely diced celery, 1 tablespoon shredded radicchio, 1 tablespoon fresh lemon juice, 2 teaspoons olive oil, ¼ teaspoon salt, and ¼ teaspoon dried tarragon. Refrigerate the mixture up to 3 hours. Bring to room temperature (about 1 hour). Spread the mixture evenly over each bread slice and serve.

**Kilocalories 228 Kc • Protein 8 Gm • Fat 5 Gm • Percent of Calories from fat 18%
• Cholesterol 0 mg • Dietary Fiber 4 Gm • Sodium 653 mg • Calcium 90 mg**

# Momos

*Momos are Tibetan dumplings. I suggest sprinkling them with tamari sauce, which is slightly thicker than soy sauce and has a richer, mellower flavor.*

½ cup diced pared potato
½ cup minced carrot
1 cup finely chopped Chinese or napa cabbage
¼ cup plain nonfat yogurt
¼ teaspoon salt

¼ teaspoon Chinese five-spice powder
¼ teaspoon chili paste
24 wonton wrappers
Tamari sauce, optional

1. Layer the potato, carrot, and cabbage in a collapsible steamer basket set over simmering water in a wide saucepan. Cover and steam 10 to 12 minutes until the potatoes are tender. Carefully remove the basket and place in the sink. Cool slightly.

2. Put the potato mixture in a medium bowl.

3. Whisk the yogurt, salt, five-spice powder, and chili paste together in a small bowl until blended. Stir into the potato mixture.

4. Spoon 1 heaping teaspoon of the mixture onto the center of each wonton wrapper. Moisten 2 edges with water, then fold over the filling to form a triangle. Press the edges together with a fork.

5. Place the wontons, in one layer, in the same collapsible steamer basket (coated with vegetable oil spray) set over simmering water in a wide saucepan. Cover and steam 5 minutes. Repeat with the remaining wontons. Remove with a flexible spatula. Serve with tamari sauce, if desired.

SERVES 4 (MAKES 24)

Kilocalories 182 Kc • Protein 7 Gm • Fat 1 Gm • Percent of calories from fat 4% • Cholesterol 5 mg • Dietary Fiber 1 Gm • Sodium 444 mg • Calcium 74 mg

# Swiss Chard and Ricotta Phyllo Packets

*I like to serve this dish with grilled chicken or fish and roasted red peppers.*

4 cups chopped Swiss chard
   leaves
½ cup sun-dried tomato bits
2 cups part-skim ricotta cheese
   (15 ounces)

½ teaspoon salt
½ teaspoon freshly ground
   pepper
12 sheets phyllo dough,
   thawed

1. Preheat the oven to 400°.

2. Place the Swiss chard in a collapsible steamer basket set over simmering water in a wide saucepan; add the tomatoes. Cover and steam 10 minutes until the chard is tender. Cool. Combine the mixture with the ricotta, salt, and pepper in a medium bowl.

3. Coat 3 layers of the phyllo dough with vegetable oil spray and stack them (keep the remaining dough covered with damp paper towels), with one long side facing you. Place a heaping ½ cup of the Swiss chard mixture into center of the stacked sheet. Fold the short ends to the center over the filling, overlapping them, then fold one long end up and the other long end down so that the filling won't leak through. Repeat with the remaining phyllo and filling.

4. Place the packets on a baking sheet coated with vegetable oil spray. Bake 20 minutes until golden. Serve immediately.

SERVES 4

**Kilocalories 309 Kc • Protein 18 Gm • Fat 7 Gm • Percent of calories from fat 19% • Cholesterol 16 mg • Dietary Fiber 4 Gm • Sodium 1026 mg • Calcium 238 mg**

# Grilled Collard-Wrapped Blackfish (Outdoor Grill)

*Blackfish is a local Long Island fish that is occasionally found along the East Coast as far north as Maine. Mahimahi or grouper is a good meaty substitute. If one collard is not large enough to cover the fish, place 2 leaves together with the ends overlapping. The collards are more tender when grilled raw rather than steamed first.*

| | |
|---|---|
| 2 large garlic cloves | ¼ teaspoon salt |
| 2 tablespoons (packed) fresh basil leaves | 4 blackfish fillets (about 5 ounces each) |
| 1 tablespoon (packed) fresh flat-leaf parsley leaves | 4 to 8 large collard leaves, thick stems removed and ribs slit an inch from base |
| 1 teaspoon fresh oregano leaves | |
| 2 tablespoon olive oil | Lemon wedges for garnish, optional |
| 1 teaspoon fresh lemon juice | |

1. Place a grill rack 5 inches from the coals and coat with vegetable oil spray. Prepare the grill following the manufacturer's instructions.

2. Chop the garlic in a small food processor. Add the basil, parsley, and oregano and mince. Add the oil, lemon juice, and salt and process until combined, scraping down the sides of the container, if necessary.

3. Coat both sides of each fillet with the garlic mixture and place in the center of a collard leaf. Fold all four sides over the mixture to form a packet. Coat the packet with vegetable oil spray.

4. Grill the fish, seam side down, over hot coals, 5 minutes on each side until opaque and firm to the touch. Serve immediately with lemon wedges, if desired.

SERVES 4

Kilocalories 288 Kc • Protein 35 Gm • Fat 14 Gm • Percent of calories from fat 43%
• Cholesterol 123 mg • Dietary Fiber 1 Gm • Sodium 284 mg • Calcium 173 mg

# Salmon Steamed in Cabbage

*Rosa Lo San Ross is a famous New York cooking teacher and cookbook author. This recipe is a favorite among her students.*

8 large napa or Chinese cabbage leaves

4 salmon steaks, ¾ inch thick (about 6 ounces each), skinned and boned

1 tablespoon white wine or vegetable broth

2 teaspoons low-sodium soy sauce

¼ cup minced scallions

1 tablespoon minced fresh ginger

2 teaspoons fresh thyme or chopped cilantro (½ teaspoon dried)

Soy sauce for garnish, optional

1. Pour 4 cups of water into a large skillet and bring to a boil. Add the cabbage leaves, cover, and steam about 1 minute until the leaves are soft and pliable. Remove and drain on paper towels.

2. Wrap the tails of the salmon around to form each steak into a circle. Place each salmon on 2 overlapping cabbage leaves.

3. Combine the wine and soy sauce in a small bowl and sprinkle over the salmon on the leaves. Top each steak with equal amounts of scallions, ginger, and thyme. Fold the leaves around the fish to form a package.

4. Place the packets in a collapsible steamer basket set over simmering water in a wide saucepan.* Cover and steam until the fish is firm to the touch and just cooked in the center, 10 to 12 minutes.

5. Remove the fish to a serving platter and sprinkle with soy sauce, if desired.

SERVES 4

*Ms. Ross suggests placing the fish on a plate that fits into a bamboo steamer basket. Cover and steam 10 to 12 minutes. If you use this method, you can pour off the juices that have accumulated on the plate into a small saucepan. Stir in 1 teaspoon cornstarch and bring to a boil, stirring until slightly thickened. Season with salt and pepper to taste and pour over the fish packages.

Kilocalories 259 Kc • Protein 35 Gm • Fat 11 Gm • Percent of calories from fat 39% • Cholesterol 93 mg • Dietary Fiber 1 Gm • Sodium 189 mg • Calcium 42 mg

# Steamed Spinach-Filled Chicken Rolls

*These tasty rolls are terrific with brown rice and snow peas stir-fried in a little dark sesame oil.*

4 5-ounce boneless, skinless chicken breast cutlets, flattened to ¼-inch thick
1½ tablespoons hoisin sauce
1 package (10 ounces) frozen chopped spinach, thawed, drained, and squeezed

8 red bell pepper strips
2 small scallions, halved lengthwise and crosswise
¼ cup reduced-sodium soy sauce

1. Brush 1 side of each cutlet with the hoisin sauce. Divide the vegetables evenly and place on one long edge of each cutlet. Roll up the chicken lengthwise and skewer with toothpicks.

2. Place the rolls in a collapsible steamer basket set over simmering water in a wide saucepan or a medium skillet. Cover and steam 12 to 15 minutes, turning occasionally, until cooked through. Lift the chicken from the steamer with tongs. Remove the toothpicks and cut each roll into 4 slices. Spoon 1 tablespoon soy sauce onto each of 4 plates. Top with the sliced chicken, cut side up.

SERVES 4

**Variation:** Steam 2 cups shredded bok choy instead of the frozen spinach. Follow the above directions, using the same steamer basket to steam the stuffed chicken rolls.

Kilocalories 317 Kc • Protein 52 Gm • Fat 7 Gm • Percent of calories from fat 20% • Cholesterol 129 mg • Dietary Fiber 3 Gm • Sodium 783 mg • Calcium 137 mg

# Sweet and Sour Stuffed Cabbage for a Crowd

*Lynn Kutner has been teaching cooking classes at the New School in Manhattan since 1974. Her stuffed cabbage, although time-consuming, is fabulous. Not bad for a Brooklyn College philosophy major!*

*Filling:*

6 medium onions (about 1½ pounds), chopped
1 tablespoon vegetable oil
2 cups tomato juice
¾ teaspoon salt
¼ teaspoon freshly ground pepper
2 large egg whites
¾ cup chopped fresh curly parsley
6 tablespoons matzo meal
3 pounds ground lean turkey

*Cabbage:*

2 to 3 heads green cabbage (6 to 7 pounds)

*Sauce:*

2¼ cups sugar
8 cups boiling water
1⅓ cups fresh lemon juice (5 to 7 lemons)
2 cans (6 ounces each) tomato paste
1 can (12 ounces) tomato sauce
½ teaspoon freshly ground pepper
¾ teaspoon Hungarian sweet paprika
Salt

1. Combine the onions, oil, and ¼ cup water in a large nonstick skillet. Cover and cook over low heat for 15 minutes. Increase the heat to medium, uncover, and cook, stirring occasionally, 15 minutes longer or until the water is absorbed.

2. Combine 1½ cups of the tomato juice with the remaining filling ingredients and half of the onions in a large bowl. Cover and refrigerate until ready to use.

3. Bring a large pot of salted water to a boil. Meanwhile, cut a circle around the core of each cabbage to loosen the leaves. Choose the largest 40 leaves, picking from both heads. Drop about 10 leaves at a time (the

amount depends on the size of your pot) into the water and boil for 4 minutes until they are pliable. Drain and cut out a little of the thick rib to make rolling the leaves easier.

4. To prepare the sauce, combine the sugar and ½ cup water in a large heavy pot. Place over high heat. Swirl the pan to dissolve the sugar but do not stir. Cover the pan for 1 minute until the sugar is completely dissolved. Wash down the sides of the pot with a pastry brush dipped in cold water. Caramelize to a medium amber color. At this point, turn off the heat or the sugar will burn. Avert your face and carefully add 2 cups of the boiling water. Stir with a wooden spoon to dissolve the caramel. Turn the heat to low and stir the mixture constantly until thoroughly dissolved. Stir in the remaining 6 cups boiling water, lemon juice, tomato paste, tomato sauce, pepper, paprika, and the reserved onions and bring to a boil. Add salt to taste and remove from the heat.

5. Preheat the oven to 425°.

6. To prepare the cabbage rolls, spoon about 2 tablespoons of the turkey mixture onto each leaf. Fold the sides over, then roll from the bottom to make a sausage-shaped package.

7. Place half of the sauce in a large roasting pan; arrange the cabbage rolls on top and cover with the remaining sauce. Cover with foil. Place the pan on a rack in the lower third of the oven. When the sauce comes to a simmer, reduce the heat to 325°. Bake 2 hours. Uncover and cool completely. Cover and refrigerate overnight. (This tastes better the next day.) To serve, place the covered pan in a 350° oven until heated through. If the sauce thickens too much, add a little warm water.

SERVES 12 (35 TO 40 ROLLS)

Kilocalories 504 Kc • Protein 27 Gm • Fat 14 Gm • Percent of calories from fat 24% • Cholesterol 108 mg • Dietary Fiber 8 Gm • Sodium 888 mg • Calcium 165 mg

# Pollack in Lettuce Packets

4 large romaine lettuce leaves
½ cup bottled clam juice
1 tablespoon distilled white
    vinegar
1 bay leaf
4 pollack fillets (about 5 ounces
    each)

½ teaspoon lemon pepper
¼ cup sour cream
¼ cup finely chopped yellow
    summer squash
¼ cup finely chopped red bell
    pepper

1. Heat ½ cup water in a large skillet over medium heat. Add the lettuce, cover, and cook 2 to 3 minutes, until limp. Remove the lettuce with a slotted spatula and place, flat side down, on paper towels to drain.

2. Add the clam juice, vinegar, and bay leaf to the water in the skillet. Bring to a simmer, covered, over low heat.

3. Place each fish fillet in the center of a lettuce leaf; sprinkle each with lemon pepper. Fold both sides of the lettuce lengthwise over the fish, then fold up the ends. Carefully place the packets, seam side down, in the liquid. Cover and cook 7 minutes. Turn the heat off and let the packets remain in the liquid for 3 minutes. Remove to a serving platter with a slotted spatula. Garnish with the sour cream, squash, and red pepper. Serve immediately.

SERVES 4

Kilocalories 231 Kc • Protein 30 Gm • Fat 10 Gm • Percent of calories from fat 42% • Cholesterol 112 mg • Dietary Fiber 1 Gm • Sodium 232 mg • Calcium 84 mg

# Roasted Red Chard and Salmon

*For a complementary side dish, combine cooked basmati rice with raisins and a tablespoon or two of pistachio nuts.*

4 salmon fillets (about 5 ounces each)

4 large red Swiss chard leaves, stems removed (spin dry)

2 tablespoons fresh lemon juice

2 teaspoons grated fresh ginger with juice

¼ teaspoon kosher or coarse salt

Freshly ground pepper

1. Preheat the oven to 400°.

2. Place each fillet in the center of a chard leaf. Sprinkle each fillet with lemon juice, gingerroot, salt, and pepper. Roll each leaf, stem end to tip, over the fillets, tucking the ends under to close, if large enough. It's O.K. if the ends aren't closed.

3. Place the packets, side by side, in an 11 × 7-inch baking pan coated with vegetable oil spray. Coat each packet with additional spray. Roast until the fish is firm to the touch and just cooked in the center, 12 to 15 minutes. Serve immediately.

SERVES 4

Kilocalories 218 Kc • Protein 29 Gm • Fat 9 Gm • Percent of calories from fat 38% • Cholesterol 78 mg • Dietary Fiber 1 Gm • Sodium 322 mg • Calcium 55 mg

# Poached Salmon Steaks with Green Sauce

*This green sauce is made with spinach and goes well with any poached or grilled fish.*

*Green Sauce:*

2 cups (packed) coarsely
    chopped fresh spinach
2 tablespoons red wine vinegar
1 hard-cooked egg
2 teaspoons vegetable oil
¼ teaspoon salt
¼ teaspoon freshly ground
    pepper

*Poaching Liquid:*

2 cups water
1 cup bottled clam juice
5 fresh flat-leaf parsley sprigs
4 peppercorns
2 ribs celery, chopped
1 bay leaf
1 teaspoon salt

4 salmon steaks, ¾ inch thick
    (about 1¾ pounds)

1. Combine all of the sauce ingredients in a blender with 3 tablespoons water. Pulse on chop, then puree, scraping down the sides of the blender, if necessary. Refrigerate until ready to use.

2. Combine all of the poaching liquid ingredients in a large skillet. Heat to boiling. Reduce the heat, cover, and simmer 5 minutes. Add the salmon and additional water to cover, if necessary. Heat to boiling. Reduce the heat and simmer, uncovered, until the fish is opaque in the center and tender, about 12 minutes.

3. Carefully remove the fish with a slotted spatula and drain on a wire rack (with paper towels underneath). Remove the skin. Cover and refrigerate at least 4 hours or overnight. Serve each steak chilled with about ¼ cup of the sauce.

SERVES 4

**Variation:** Green Mayo Sauce: ½ cup (packed) coarsely chopped fresh spinach, ¼ cup light mayonnaise, 2 teaspoons Worcestershire sauce, 2 teaspoons brandy, 1 teaspoon tomato paste, ¼ teaspoon dry mustard, and a few drops of Tabasco sauce. Combine all of the ingredients in a small food processor and process until the spinach is pureed. Spread a heaping table-spoonful of the sauce over each steak. Makes ⅓ cup.

**Kilocalories 329 Kc • Protein 42 Gm • Fat 16 Gm • Percent of calories from fat 46% • Cholesterol 162 mg • Dietary Fiber 1 Gm • Sodium 271 mg • Calcium 59 mg**

# Spinach Sushi

*Sushi rice is a short-grained rice that gets sticky when cooked. It's sold in Asian supermarkets.*

2 tablespoons low-sodium soy sauce, plus additional for dipping (optional)
1 tablespoon dark sesame oil
1 tablespoon hoisin sauce
2 seaweed sheets (nori), toasted (follow package instructions)
2 cups cooked white rice (preferably sushi rice)

2 teaspoons grated fresh ginger
1 cup fresh spinach leaves
1 cup roasted peppers, cut into long thin slices
12 blanched snow peas for garnish, optional

1. Combine the soy sauce, oil, and hoisin sauce in a small bowl.

2. Place each seaweed sheet on wax paper. Brush each sheet lightly with the soy mixture. (Do not soak the sheets or they won't roll properly.) Reserve the remaining soy sauce mixture.

3. Combine the rice and ginger in a medium bowl. Spread 1 cup of this mixture evenly on each sheet to within ½ inch of the edges. Sprinkle with the remaining soy mixture. Place the spinach leaves, then the pepper slices over the rice.

4. Lightly roll up, jelly-roll fashion, using the wax paper to lift the sheet and gently roll. Wrap each roll in the wax paper and place, seam side down, on a flat surface in the refrigerator. Refrigerate at least 3 hours or until firm.

5. To serve, cut each roll into 8 equal pieces with a serrated knife. Place 4 pieces of sushi on each of 4 serving plates. Garnish the plate with the snow pea pods in the shape of a fan and serve with soy sauce, if desired.

SERVES 4

Kilocalories 189 Kc • Protein 5 Gm • Fat 4 Gm • Percent of calories from fat 18% • Cholesterol 0 mg • Dietary Fiber 2 Gm • Sodium 320 mg • Calcium 25 mg

# Grilled Peppered Shark and Romaine (Outdoor Grill)

*The romaine lettuce is actually steamed in foil on the grill. Serve with ripe herbed tomatoes and paper-thin slices of raw zucchini, and there's no need to go near the stove during the hot summer months.*

3 tablespoons whole black peppercorns

1¼ pounds shark steak, about ¾ inch thick

1 medium head romaine lettuce

2 tablespoons distilled white vinegar

2 teaspoons extra-virgin olive oil

¼ teaspoon kosher or coarse salt

1. Crush the peppercorns with a pestle. Press into both sides of the shark steak. Cover and let it stand at room temperature for 30 minutes.

2. Place the grill rack 5 inches from the coals and coat with vegetable oil spray. Prepare the grill following manufacturer's instructions.

3. Cut the romaine lettuce in half lengthwise. Add the vinegar to a sinkful of water and soak the romaine in the water-vinegar mixture for 20 minutes. Carefully remove any dirt that remains between the leaves, without breaking the leaves from the base. Remove from the water and drain, cut side down, on paper towels.

4. Coat both sides of the lettuce with vegetable oil spray. Wrap each half in foil and grill over medium-hot coals about 15 minutes, turning once.

5. Meanwhile, grill the fish 4 to 5 minutes on each side or until it is done to your liking. Cut into 4 pieces.

6. Remove the foil from the lettuce, cut each piece in half crosswise, and place on a serving platter. Drizzle with the oil and sprinkle with the salt. Add the fish to the platter and serve immediately.

SERVES 4

Kilocalories 221 Kc • Protein 31 Gm • Fat 9 Gm • Percent of calories from fat 37% • Cholesterol 72 mg • Dietary Fiber 2 Gm • Sodium 263 mg • Calcium 79 mg

# 10
# Rustic Breads and Other Savories

There's nothing better than the aroma of freshly baked breads, rolls, and muffins unless, of course, it's the smell of pizza, focaccia, or savory tarts wafting from your own kitchen oven. This chapter has them all.

If you've always wanted to be a baker but were hesitant to try, this chapter is for you. You'll need to know some basic terms before launching into the world of yeast, so check the following definitions and suggestions before you begin.

1. Water: Some recipes call for warm water (105 to 115°). If you have a thermometer, fine. If not, the hand test is very accurate. Run the hot water faucet, and place your fingers under the running water. When the water feels very warm but not too hot to the touch, it's about the right temperature.

2. Proofing the yeast: A fancy term for a simple technique. All it means is that you fill a bowl with warm water, sprinkle the yeast on top, and add a pinch of sugar. It's a good test. If the yeast, which normally gobbles up sugar, doesn't foam and

bubble, it's past its prime. Throw it out and start again or your bread will be like lead.

3. Kneading: This can be done by machine (food processor or heavy duty mixer) or by hand. Kneading dough is essential to the formation of gluten, the protein component of wheat flour that gives structure to the bread. Think of gluten as a large spider web with trampoline capabilities; if you jump on it you'll bounce around because the fiber is strong.

   To knead by hand, simply press down on the dough with the heels of both hands (although I often use one hand), pushing away from your body. Then fold the dough toward you and give it a quarter turn. The process is repeated until the dough is no longer sticky but smooth and elastic. This usually takes 8 to 10 minutes. At this point, if you poke a finger into the dough gently, the dough will spring back lightly.

4. Doneness: The hallowed test for doneness is to tap on the bottom of the bread. If it sounds hollow, it's done. This is O.K. for breads baked on a sheet. Personally, I don't like turning a steaming hot bread out of the loaf pan to do this test. An easier, yet equally reliable, test for doneness is to insert a thermometer into the center of the bread. When it registers 200° it's done.

5. Freezing: Fresh bread is wonderful and I prefer to eat it the day that it's made, but it may be frozen. Always completely cool the bread or rolls on a wire rack first. Wrap the cooled bread in foil; then place it in an airtight sealable plastic bag. Label and freeze.

   Raw dough may also be frozen and then defrosted, overnight, in the refrigerator. I place it in a sealable plastic bag, remove the air, and freeze. When it defrosts, it has room to expand. The texture of the dough, however, changes slightly. I find the dough becomes more elastic and is harder to roll or stretch. Sometimes, in the case of focaccia, I bake the bread, topping and all, and freeze it, wrapped in foil. When I'm ready to serve it, I place it in a 350° oven for about 20 minutes until it is heated through.

6. Methods for Bread Making: Machine and hand methods are interchangeable. There are many recipes using both methods, so the choice is yours.

# Baked Pita Bread and Beet Greens

*Ackawi is semisoft cheese that's a cross between mozzarella and feta cheese. If you can't find it in your supermarket, I recommend using feta cheese for this small meal with "zip."*

2 (7-inch) pocketless pita breads, homemade if desired (page 335)
2 cups (packed) chopped beet greens
¼ teaspoon freshly ground pepper

8 kalamata olives, pitted and chopped
¼ cup grated Ackawi cheese
2 teaspoons olive oil

1. Preheat the oven to 450°.
2. Place the pita breads on a baking sheet. Top with the greens, pepper, olives, and cheese. Drizzle with the oil. Bake 10 minutes and serve.

SERVES 2

Kilocalories 305 Kc • Protein 13 Gm • Fat 11 Gm • Percent of calories from fat 32% • Cholesterol 12 mg • Dietary Fiber 4 Gm • Sodium 986 mg • Calcium 315 mg

# Homemade Pocketless Pita Bread with Wilted Salad Greens

*These pita breads are like puffy pizza. Any steamed or sautéed greens would make a delicious topping. Even raw salad greens with an exotic dressing—cumin or beet—would be delicious, but would require a knife and fork.*

*Dough:*

1 cup warm water (105 to 115°)
1 package active dry yeast
½ teaspoon sugar
1½ tablespoons olive oil
2 cups all-purpose flour
¾ cup whole wheat flour
¼ teaspoon salt

*Salad:*

12 cups mesclun (about 6 ounces)
1 tablespoon sherry vinegar
¼ teaspoon kosher or coarse salt

1. To prepare the bread, place the water in a medium bowl; sprinkle with the yeast and sugar. Let the mixture stand 10 minutes, until bubbly. Stir in ½ tablespoon of the oil, the all-purpose flour, ½ cup of the whole wheat flour, and the salt. Stir until a dough forms. Turn onto a lightly floured surface and knead 8 to 10 minutes, adding the remaining ¼ cup whole wheat flour gradually until the dough is smooth and elastic. Place the dough in a large bowl coated with vegetable oil spray. Coat the top of the dough with additional spray and cover the bowl tightly with plastic wrap. Let it rise in a warm place about 1 hour, until doubled in size.

2. Preheat the oven to 500°.

3. While the dough is rising, heat the remaining 1 tablespoon of oil in a large nonstick skillet over medium-low heat. Add the mesclun and sprinkle with the vinegar. Cover and cook 1 minute. Uncover, stir, and remove from the heat. Cool.

4. Punch down the dough and divide it into 4 equal pieces. Shape each piece into a disk and flatten. Roll each disk into a 7-inch circle. Place on a baking sheet coated with vegetable oil spray (I was able to fit all four on

one sheet). Bake 10 minutes until puffy and browned. Top each pizza with the greens and sprinkle with the kosher salt.

SERVES 4

**Kilocalories 382 Kc • Protein 12 Gm • Fat 7 Gm • Percent of calories from fat 15% • Cholesterol 0 mg • Dietary Fiber 7 Gm • Sodium 313 mg • Calcium 164 mg**

# Italian Griddle Bread (Piadina)

*Emilia Romagna is a region in Italy famous for Reggiano-Parmigiano cheese. Not so famous* piadina *is a wonderful flat bread made with lard.* Piadine *are sold at large street stands and are filled with either greens or cheese and folded to make a portable sandwich—typical Italian street food. On one of our trips to Italy, we bought a variety of these sandwiches, a tub of olives, and some regional cheeses and wine. Along with our friends, we happily lunched on the terrace of our hotel room. That afternoon's small feast is a fond memory.*

*Filling:*

1½ tablespoons olive oil
3 garlic cloves, minced
2 bunches beet greens (about 2 pounds), trimmed and chopped
1 teaspoon salt
¼ teaspoon freshly ground pepper

*Piadina Dough:*

2 cups unbleached all-purpose flour
¼ teaspoon salt
¼ teaspoon baking soda
2 tablespoons vegetable shortening
½ cup warm water

1. To prepare the filling, heat the oil in a Dutch oven over medium-low heat. Add the garlic and cook about 30 seconds or until it just barely browns. Add the wet greens, salt, pepper, and ¼ cup water. Cover and cook, stirring occasionally, for 10 minutes.

2. Preheat the oven to 200°.

3. To prepare the bread, place the flour, salt, and baking soda in a food processor fitted with the steel blade. Pulse once or twice to combine. Add the vegetable shortening and process for 10 seconds. With the machine running, add the warm water through the feed tube and process about 10 seconds or until the dough looks like large crumbs; the dough should not form a ball.

4. Turn the dough onto a flat surface and press into a ball. Knead 2 or 3 times until it holds together. (The dough will be elastic, but not sticky.) Divide the dough into 6 equal pieces and roll each into a ball. Roll each ball into a 7-inch circle.

5. Coat a nonstick griddle or skillet with vegetable oil spray. Heat over medium-high heat. Cook each piadina about 30 seconds on each side until lightly browned and speckled. Cover with foil and place in the oven until ready to serve (up to 30 minutes.)

6. To serve, reheat the greens; drain. Arrange about a heaping ½ cup of greens in the center of each piadina. Fold in half and serve immediately.

MAKES 6 BREADS

**Variation:** For a less traditional and heartier sandwich, add 1½ cups julienned cooked beets and ½ cup shredded part-skim mozzarella. Divide evenly over the greens and fold.

Kilocalories 316 Kc • Protein 13 Gm • Fat 9 Gm • Percent of calories from fat 23% • Cholesterol 0 mg • Dietary Fiber 12 Gm • Sodium 1378 mg • Calcium 447 mg

# Collard/Buttermilk Biscuits

3 cups all-purpose flour
¼ cup sugar
1½ teaspoons baking soda
1 teaspoon baking powder
¾ teaspoon salt
1½ cups low-fat buttermilk

⅓ cup vegetable oil
2 large eggs
1 package (10 ounces)
 frozen collard greens,
 thawed, drained, and
 squeezed

1. Preheat the oven to 400°F. Coat sixteen 2¾-inch muffin cups with vegetable oil spray. (These biscuits will stick to paper liners.)

2. Combine the flour, sugar, baking soda, baking powder, and salt in a large bowl. Whisk the buttermilk, oil, and eggs in a 4-cup measure. Pour the buttermilk mixture into the dry ingredients. Stir until just blended. Add the greens.

3. Turn the batter into the prepared pan, filling each cup about ¾ full. Bake 20 minutes or until a toothpick inserted in the center comes out clean. Cool in the pan on a rack for 10 minutes. Serve or cool completely and freeze in a sealable plastic bag.

MAKES 16 BISCUITS

**Variation:** Add ¼ cup imitation bacon bits and ½ teaspoon freshly ground black pepper for a truly southern treat.

Kilocalories 162 Kc • Protein 4 Gm • Fat 6 Gm • Percent of calories from fat 31% • Cholesterol 27 mg • Dietary Fiber 1 Gm • Sodium 293 mg • Calcium 102 mg

# Collard and Chicken Sausage Biscuit Pie

*This is my first biscuit pie. Although the crust is not flaky, like homemade pastry dough, it sure is easier and quicker to prepare.*

1½ tablespoons vegetable oil
2 garlic cloves, minced
1 pound chicken sausage, cut
    into 1-inch pieces

8 ounces fresh collards, trimmed
    and chopped
½ teaspoon salt
2½ cups Bisquick

1. Preheat the oven to 450°.

2. Coat a large nonstick skillet with vegetable oil spray. Add ½ tablespoon of the oil and place over medium heat. When the oil is hot, add the garlic and sausage. Cook, stirring frequently, 3 minutes until the chicken is no longer pink. Top with the collards, cover, and cook, stirring occasionally, 5 minutes until the collards are wilted and tender. Remove from the heat and stir in the salt and the remaining 1 tablespoon oil. Cool.

3. Coat a 9-inch pie pan with vegetable oil spray.

4. Combine the Bisquick with ½ cup cold water. Stir with a fork until a fairly stiff dough forms. Shape into 2 balls, one slightly larger than the other. On a lightly floured surface, roll the larger portion into a 10-inch circle. Fold in half and carefully place in the center of the prepared pan. Unfold, and gently ease into the pan and trim the edges. Spoon the collard mixture into the pie shell.

5. Roll the remaining ball into a 9-inch circle and place on top of the pie. Press the edges together to seal and flute the dough by pressing the edges with a fork or between your fingers. Bake about 20 minutes until the pie is golden. Let it stand 5 minutes before serving.

SERVES 6

Kilocalories 367 Kc • Protein 17 Gm • Fat 18 Gm • Percent of calories from fat 43% • Cholesterol 47 mg • Dietary Fiber 2 Gm • Sodium 1506 mg • Calcium 129 mg

# Swiss Cabbage Pie

*This unusual savory pie is adapted from a recipe by my good friend and fellow cookbook author, Lyn Stallworth, who lives in Brooklyn, New York.*

2 tablespoons vegetable oil
2 pounds cabbage, shredded
(about 8 cups)
2 tablespoons all-purpose flour
2 tablespoons snipped fresh dill
½ teaspoon salt
½ teaspoon freshly ground black
pepper

1 cup evaporated skimmed
milk
2 large eggs
2 egg whites
½ cup shredded Swiss cheese,
optional
1 pound frozen bread dough,
thawed

1. Preheat the oven to 350°.

2. Heat the oil in a Dutch oven over medium heat. Stir in the cabbage, flour, dill, salt, and pepper; cover and cook 5 to 8 minutes until softened, stirring occasionally.

3. Whisk the milk, eggs, and egg whites together in a medium bowl; add the cheese, if desired. Reduce the heat and add the egg mixture to the Dutch oven. Cook for 3 to 4 minutes, stirring frequently. Cool.

4. Place the defrosted dough in the middle of a 9-inch pie pan. Stretch to fit, folding the edges over the rim. Pour the cabbage mixture into the pie crust and bake for about 1 hour or until the filling is set and the crust is golden brown. Let the pie stand for 5 minutes before serving.

SERVES 8

Kilocalories 267 Kc • Protein 12 Gm • Fat 7 Gm • Percent of calories from fat 23%
• Cholesterol 54 mg • Dietary Fiber 4 Gm • Sodium 563 mg • Calcium 199 mg

# Swiss Chard and Ricotta Calzone

*Friends are often invited to my house for tasting dinners. The purpose is criticism—good and bad—for newly developed recipes. One group tasted a bunch of pizzas and raved until they tasted this calzone. This simple, quick stuffed bread won the Golden Whisk Award that night.*

1 pound frozen pizza dough
4 cups chopped red Swiss chard
 leaves (wet)
2 cups part-skim ricotta cheese
½ teaspoon dried basil

½ teaspoon salt
½ teaspoon freshly ground
 pepper
¼ teaspoon garlic
 powder

1. Defrost the dough according to the package directions.

2. Preheat the oven to 450°.

3. Place the chard in a saucepan. Cover and cook over low heat for 5 minutes. Remove, drain, squeeze, and cool. Combine with the ricotta, basil, salt, pepper, and garlic powder in a medium bowl.

4. Roll the dough on a floured surface to a 10-inch circle. Spoon the filling on one half, leaving a 1-inch border around the edges. Fold the other side of the dough over the filling and crimp the edges together to seal.

5. Place on a baking sheet coated with vegetable oil spray. Bake 30 to 35 minutes until browned. Let the calzone stand 5 minutes. Slice and serve.

SERVES 4

Kilocalories 409 Kc • Protein 23 Gm • Fat 7 Gm • Percent of calories from fat 16%
• Cholesterol 16 mg • Dietary Fiber 9 Gm • Sodium 1232 mg • Calcium 225 mg

# Crustless Mustard Green Pie

*This may be served as a side dish or a light main dish.*

1 cup chopped onion
¼ cup low-sodium chicken broth
  or water
2 packages (10 ounces each)
  frozen chopped mustard
  greens, thawed, drained, and
  squeezed
2 large eggs

2 egg whites
1½ cups evaporated skimmed
  milk
⅓ cup low-fat shredded Swiss
  cheese
½ teaspoon salt
½ teaspoon freshly ground
  pepper

1. Preheat the oven to 350°.

2. Combine the onion and broth in a medium skillet. Cover and cook over medium heat 3 minutes. Uncover and cook 2 minutes longer, until the liquid is absorbed. Remove from the heat.

3. Stir the mustard greens into the onion in the skillet. Spoon into a 10-inch pie plate coated with vegetable oil spray.

4. Whisk the eggs and egg whites together in a 4-cup measure; add the milk, cheese, salt, and pepper and whisk to combine. Pour into the greens mixture and stir to combine. Bake 30 minutes or until the center is almost set. Cool on a wire rack 10 minutes. Cut and serve.

SERVES 4

Kilocalories 227 Kc • Protein 22 Gm • Fat 7 Gm • Percent of calories from fat 25%
• Cholesterol 119 mg • Dietary Fiber 5 Gm • Sodium 604 mg • Calcium 642 mg

# Collard Pumpkin Rolls

*This is a tasty way to use those Halloween pumpkins.*

½ cup warm skim milk (105 to 115°)
1 package active dry yeast
½ cup pumpkin puree
1 tablespoon (packed) dark brown sugar
¾ teaspoon salt
⅛ teaspoon ground ginger
⅛ teaspoon ground cinnamon
2½ to 3 cups all-purpose flour
½ package (10 ounces) frozen chopped collard greens, thawed, drained, and squeezed
1 tablespoon skim milk
½ teaspoon poppy seeds

1. Combine the warm milk and yeast in a large bowl. Let it stand 10 minutes until bubbly. Stir in the pumpkin, sugar, salt, ginger, and cinnamon. Add 2½ cups of the flour and the collards, stirring with a fork to combine.

2. Knead the dough on a lightly floured surface for 8 to 10 minutes, adding more flour, if necessary, until smooth and elastic.

3. Place the dough in a large bowl coated with vegetable oil spray, turning to coat. Cover with plastic wrap and let it rise in a warm place for 1 hour or until double in size.

4. Punch down the dough; place on a lightly floured surface. Divide into 12 pieces. Tuck the ends under to form smooth balls. Arrange on a baking sheet coated with vegetable oil spray, in a circle, with the rolls touching each other. Cover loosely with a towel and let them rise until nearly double in size, about 30 minutes.

5. Preheat the oven to 375°.

6. Brush the tops of the rolls with the milk and sprinkle with the poppy seeds. Bake 25 to 30 minutes or until lightly browned. Cool the rolls on a wire rack.

MAKES 12 ROLLS

Kilocalories 113 Kc • Protein 4 Gm • Fat 0 Gm • Percent of calories from fat 3% • Cholesterol 0 mg • Dietary Fiber 2 Gm • Sodium 159 mg • Calcium 73 mg

# Multigrain and Greens Bread

*Although I've used an electric mixer for this recipe, it may be done in a food processor using the plastic dough blade or by hand. Just follow another recipe in this chapter that uses one of those methods.*

1½ cups skim milk
¼ cup honey
1 package active dry yeast
3 to 3½ cups all-purpose
    flour
½ cup whole wheat flour
½ cup rolled oats

2 tablespoons whole grain
    amaranth (or millet)
1½ teaspoons salt
1 package (10 ounces) frozen
    chopped greens (your choice),
    thawed, drained, and squeezed
¼ cup toasted sesame seeds

1. Combine the milk and honey in a small saucepan over low heat. Heat until the thermometer registers 105 to 115°. Remove from the heat and sprinkle with the yeast. Let it stand for 10 minutes until bubbly.

2. Combine 3 cups of the all-purpose flour, the whole wheat flour, oats, amaranth, and salt in the large bowl of an electric mixer fitted with the dough hook. Add the milk mixture and mix at low speed until a dough forms, about 2 minutes. Increase the mixer speed to medium and add the greens and ½ cup more of the all-purpose flour. Beat 10 minutes or until soft and pliable.

3. Turn the dough out onto a lightly floured surface. Knead about 3 minutes until smooth and elastic, adding additional flour, if necessary. Place the dough in a bowl coated with vegetable oil spray; turn to coat. Cover it with plastic wrap and let it rise in a warm place until double in size, about 1 hour.

4. Punch down the dough and turn onto a lightly floured surface. Roll out the dough to a 10-inch circle and sprinkle with the sesame seeds. Fold the dough over the seeds and knead to incorporate the seeds. Shape the dough into an oval loaf and place in a 9 × 5-inch loaf pan coated with vegetable oil spray. Cover with plastic wrap and let it rise in a warm place until double in size, about 45 minutes.

5. While the dough is rising a second time, preheat the oven to 350°.

Bake for 45 to 55 minutes until the bread is golden. Remove from the pan and cool on a wire rack.

MAKES 1 LOAF (16 SLICES)

Kilocalories 173 Kc • Protein 6 Gm • Fat 2 Gm • Percent of calories from fat 9% • Cholesterol 0 mg • Dietary Fiber 2 Gm • Sodium 247 mg • Calcium 109 mg

# Easy Watercress Biscuits

1 can (8 ounce) refrigerator biscuits

½ cup grated sharp Cheddar cheese (2 ounces)

¼ cup finely chopped watercress

2 teaspoons sesame seeds

1. Preheat the oven to 400°.
2. Pat each biscuit to a 3½-inch circle on a lightly floured surface. Pinch the edge to make a rim.
3. Combine the cheese and watercress in a small bowl. Spoon the mixture onto the biscuits. Sprinkle the edges of the biscuits with sesame seeds. Place on an ungreased baking sheet. Bake 7 to 10 minutes until golden. Serve immediately.

SERVES 4

Kilocalories 227 Kc • Protein 7 Gm • Fat 7 Gm • Percent of calories from fat 29% • Cholesterol 11 mg • Dietary Fiber 0 Gm • Sodium 972 mg • Calcium 97 mg

# Spinach Corn Bread

*Corn bread is always good with stew or gumbo. It there are any leftovers, sprinkle them with a little cheese and place in the toaster oven for a few minutes.*

1 cup all-purpose flour
1 cup yellow cornmeal
1 tablespoon baking powder
1 teaspoon salt
⅛ teaspoon ground red pepper
1 cup skim milk

2 tablespoons vegetable oil
1 large egg, lightly beaten
½ package (10 ounces) frozen
    chopped spinach, thawed,
    drained, and squeezed
¼ cup finely chopped onion

1. Preheat the oven to 400°.

2. Combine the flour, cornmeal, baking powder, salt, and pepper in a medium bowl.

3. Whisk the milk, oil, and egg together in a 2-cup measure. Pour it into the dry ingredients and stir lightly. Add the spinach and onion to the mixture; stir to combine.

4. Pour the mixture into an 8-inch square pan coated with vegetable oil spray. Bake until a toothpick inserted in the center comes out clean, about 20 minutes. Cool on a rack in the pan for 10 minutes. Loosen the edges and remove from the pan. Cut into 6 equal pieces and serve.

SERVES 6

Kilocalories 226 Kc • Protein 7 Gm • Fat 6 Gm • Percent of calories from fat 25% • Cholesterol 36 mg • Dietary Fiber 3 Gm • Sodium 647 mg • Calcium 195 mg

# Stuffed Blue Corn Bread

*Alice Murray, an interfaith minister and healer, gave me a bag of blue cornmeal before she moved West. She and her husband, John, have no idea where in the West they will settle. They're letting their spirit guide them to the right place. Wherever it is, I know I'll always have a supply of blue cornmeal. The following recipe, like blue cornmeal, is not traditional—it's more vegetable, less bready, and the color of a blue spruce.*

1 package (10 ounces) frozen kale, thawed, drained, and squeezed

1 cup frozen baby lima beans, drained and patted dry

½ cup shredded low-fat Cheddar cheese (about 2 ounces)

1 jalapeño pepper, seeded and minced

½ teaspoon salt

2 cups blue cornmeal

1 teaspoon baking soda

¾ cup milk

3 tablespoons vegetable oil

1 large egg

1. Preheat the oven to 350°.

2. Combine the kale, lima beans, cheese, jalapeño, and salt in a medium bowl. Set aside.

3. Combine the cornmeal and baking soda in a second medium bowl.

4. Whisk the milk, oil, and egg together in a 2-cup measure. Pour into the dry ingredients and stir to combine.

5. Pour half of the cornmeal batter into an 8-inch square baking pan coated with vegetable oil spray. Top evenly with the kale mixture. Drizzle the remaining batter over the vegetables. Bake 25 minutes or until a toothpick inserted in the center comes out clean. Let the bread stand for 15 minutes on a wire rack before cutting into 6 pieces.

SERVES 6

Kilocalories 295 Kc • Protein 11 Gm • Fat 11 Gm • Percent of calories from fat 32% • Cholesterol 41 mg • Dietary Fiber 5 Gm • Sodium 587 mg • Calcium 193 mg

# Pizza with Smoked Mozzarella and Arugula

*This is basically a salad on a pizza. It has a wonderfully smoky flavor and is one of my favorites.*

*Dough:*

½ cup warm water (105 to 115°)
1 package active dry yeast
½ teaspoon sugar
1½ cups all-purpose flour, plus
   additional for kneading
½ teaspoon salt

*Topping:*

¼ cup grated Parmesan cheese
½ cup cubed smoked mozzarella
   (about 2 ounces)
2 cups coarsely chopped arugula
Kosher or coarse salt and freshly
   ground pepper

1. To prepare the dough, combine the water, yeast, and sugar in a medium bowl. Let it stand for 10 minutes until foamy.

2. Stir in the flour and salt until a soft mass forms. Turn onto a floured surface and knead 8 to 10 minutes, adding more flour if necessary, until the dough is smooth and elastic. Place in a large bowl coated with vegetable oil spray; turn to coat. Cover with plastic wrap and let it rise for 1 hour.

3. Preheat the oven to 500°.

4. Punch down the dough; place in the center of a 12-inch pizza pan coated with vegetable oil spray. Stretch to fit the pan. Cover with a towel and let it rise for 30 minutes. Sprinkle the dough evenly with the Parmesan cheese, then the mozzarella. Bake 10 to 12 minutes until the edges are lightly browned.

5. Top with the arugula and sprinkle with salt and pepper to taste. Serve immediately.

SERVES 4

Kilocalories 248 Kc • Protein 12 Gm • Fat 5 Gm • Percent of calories from fat 19% • Cholesterol 14 mg • Dietary Fiber 2 Gm • Sodium 456 mg • Calcium 232 mg

# Whole Wheat Pizza with Spinach and Feta

¾ cup warm water (105 to 115°)
1 package active dry yeast
½ teaspoon sugar
1 cup whole wheat flour
1 cup all-purpose flour
½ teaspoon salt

*Topping:*

½ cup sun-dried tomatoes
6 cups chopped fresh
   spinach
¼ teaspoon salt
⅓ cup crumbled feta cheese with
   black pepper
1 tablespoon olive oil

1. Combine the water, yeast, and sugar in the bowl of a food processor fitted with the steel blade. Let it stand 10 minutes until bubbly.

2. Add both kinds of flour and the salt and pulse a few times to combine. Process 40 seconds (to knead) until a ball forms.

3. Remove the dough from the food processor and knead by hand 1 minute on a floured surface, adding more flour if it is sticky. Place in a large bowl coated with vegetable oil spray, turning to coat. Cover with plastic wrap and let it rise for 1 hour or until double in size.

4. To prepare the topping, combine the tomatoes in a small bowl with very hot water to cover. Let them stand for 10 minutes; drain and chop.

5. Place the spinach in a saucepan. Cover and cook over low heat 5 minutes, until wilted. Remove, drain, and squeeze. Cool.

6. Preheat the oven to 450°. Place the dough in the center of a 12-inch pizza pan coated with vegetable oil spray. Stretch to fit the pan. Cover with a towel and let it rise for 30 minutes. Top with the spinach and sun-dried tomatoes. Sprinkle with salt and then the cheese. Drizzle with the oil. Bake about 25 minutes until the crust is browned.

SERVES 6

Kilocalories 229 Kc • Protein 10 Gm • Fat 6 Gm • Percent of calories from fat 23%
• Cholesterol 12 mg • Dietary Fiber 5 Gm • Sodium 588 mg • Calcium 160 mg

# Pizza with Escarole à la Charles

*Although I learned about a biga (starter) for tastier breads from cookbook author Carol Field, it was Charles Scicolone who added it to pizza dough. After a trip to Naples, Charles became obsessed with making pizza. In fact, he made it almost every day for weeks until his pizza tasted just like the "real" Neopolitan pizza. Thanks, Charles, for a great idea.*

*Biga: Makes 2 cups*

**1 cup warm water (105 to 115°)**
**¼ teaspoon active dry yeast**

**2½ cups unbleached all-purpose flour**

Combine the water and yeast in a medium bowl. Let it stand for 10 minutes until creamy (there's not enough yeast to really bubble up.) Stir in the flour and spoon the mixture into another bowl, coated with vegetable oil spray. Cover with plastic wrap and let it rise in a cool place for 8 to 24 hours. Refrigerate up to one week or freeze in 1 cup increments. To defrost, let the dough stand at room temperature about 3 hours or until bubbly again.

*Pizza:*

**½ cup warm water (105 to 115°)**
**1 package active dry yeast**
**½ teaspoon sugar**
**1 cup biga**
**1 tablespoon olive oil**
**2 cups unbleached all-purpose flour, plus additional for kneading if necessary**
**½ teaspoon salt**

*Topping:*

**1 head escarole (about 1½ pounds), trimmed and chopped**
**¼ cup currants or raisins**
**1 tablespoon pignoli nuts**
**2 tablespoons olive oil**
**½ teaspoon kosher or coarse salt**
**Freshly ground pepper**
**Slivered pepato cheese (black peppercorn cheese) for garnish, optional**

1. To make the dough, combine the water, yeast, and sugar in the bowl of a food processor fitted with the steel blade. Let it stand for 10 minutes until bubbly. Add the biga and oil, then the flour and salt. Pulse a few times to combine. Process 40 seconds (to knead) until a ball forms.

2. Remove the dough from the food processor and knead by hand for 1 minute on a floured surface, adding more flour if the dough is too sticky. Place in a large bowl coated with vegetable oil spray, turning to coat. Cover with plastic wrap and let it rise for 1 hour or until double in size.

3. Turn the dough onto a 12-inch pizza pan and spread it to fit the pan. Cover with a towel while preparing the topping.

4. Preheat the oven to 500°.

5. To prepare the topping, combine the wet escarole and currants in a large saucepan. Cover and cook over medium heat for 10 to 12 minutes, stirring occasionally, until wilted. Drain and cool in a colander.

6. Spread the escarole mixture to within ½ inch of the edge of the dough. Sprinkle with the pignoli nuts. Drizzle with the oil, sprinkle with the salt, and season with pepper to taste. Top with the cheese, if desired. Bake 18 to 20 minutes until browned and crisp.

Remove from the pan and cool on a rack for 5 minutes before slicing.

SERVES 6

**Variation:** Savoy Cabbage, Onion, and "Sour Cream" Pizza: Combine 4 cups shredded savoy cabbage and 2 cups thinly sliced onion with 1 tablespoon olive oil in a large nonstick skillet. Cover and cook over low heat 15 minutes, stirring occasionally. Uncover, turn the heat to medium-high, and cook 3 minutes, stirring until lightly browned. Remove from the heat and stir in ⅓ cup nonfat sour cream. Cool slightly. Spread on the dough and sprinkle with salt and pepper. Bake, following the above instructions. (This dough is thick and delicious. There's enough dough, however, to make 2 thinner pizzas; just adjust the baking time.)

Kilocalories 261 Kc • Protein 7 Gm • Fat 8 Gm • Percent of calories from fat 28% • Cholesterol 0 mg • Dietary Fiber 6 Gm • Sodium 414 mg • Calcium 111 mg

# Focaccia with Onions and Swiss Chard

*This recipe was a favorite of my students when I taught at the New School in Manhattan. It's low in fat, about 1 gram per slice, but it's about 100 calories a slice. You may wonder why this dough rises in the refrigerator overnight. The slow rise acts like a* biga, *developing more flavor. But the dough becomes more elastic and is harder to roll out. The added patience is worth the effort. The entire bread may be made, completely cooled, wrapped in foil, and frozen up to one week. When ready to serve just pop into a 350° oven until heated through.*

1½ cups warm water (105 to 115°)
1 package active dry yeast
1 teaspoon sugar
1 tablespoon extra-virgin olive oil
4 to 4½ cups unbleached all-purpose flour
1 teaspoon salt

*Topping:*

4 cups thinly sliced onion
3 teaspoons extra-virgin olive oil
2 teaspoons sugar
3 cups chopped Swiss chard leaves (wet)
½ teaspoon kosher or coarse salt
Freshly ground pepper

1. To prepare the dough, combine ½ cup of the water and yeast in a large bowl; sprinkle with the sugar. Let it stand for 10 minutes until bubbly. Stir in the oil and the remaining 1 cup water.

2. Add 4 cups of the flour and the salt; stir to form a soft dough.

3. Turn out the dough onto a lightly floured surface. Knead until it is smooth and elastic and the dough springs back when lightly poked with a finger, about 10 minutes. Add the remaining ½ cup flour, as needed, if the dough feels sticky. Place the dough in a floured, gallon-size sealable plastic bag. Refrigerate overnight until double in size.

4. To prepare the topping, combine the onion, 2 teaspoons of the oil, and the sugar in a large nonstick skillet. Cover and cook over low heat 15 minutes. Turn the heat to medium-high and add the wet Swiss chard. Cook until the onion is lightly browned and the chard is wilted, stirring frequently, 5 to 10 minutes.

5. Roll the dough out on a lightly floured surface. (Have some fun and

hold it and let it hang and stretch, like they do in pizza parlors.) Place the dough on a 15 × 10-inch jelly-roll pan coated with vegetable oil spray. Keep pressing and stretching the dough until it fits to the corners of the pan. Cover with a clean kitchen towel and let it rise 45 minutes.

6. Preheat the oven to 450°.

7. Spoon the onion mixture onto the dough, spreading it evenly (it's easier to use your hands). Drizzle with the remaining 1 teaspoon oil, sprinkle with the salt, and season with pepper to taste. Bake 10 minutes. Reduce the heat to 400° and bake 20 minutes longer until crisp and browned. Cut into 3 × 2-inch slices.

MAKES 25 SLICES

**Kilocalories 98 Kc • Protein 3 Gm • Fat 1 Gm • Percent of calories from fat 12% • Cholesterol 0 mg • Dietary Fiber 1 Gm • Sodium 169 mg • Calcium 36 mg**

# Batter Bread Chicory Pizza

*This is really a quick bread. Baking powder is used instead of yeast, which makes this light and cakey rather than chewy. It's a great substitute for potatoes or rice as a side dish. As a main dish, I'd serve this pizza with a tomato or fennel and orange salad, maybe even a warm bean salad.*

*Batter:*

2 cups all-purpose flour
1 tablespoon baking powder
1 teaspoon dried oregano
¼ teaspoon salt
¼ teaspoon freshly ground
  pepper
2 large eggs
2 egg whites

¾ cup skim milk
1 tablespoon olive oil

*Topping:*

4 cups finely chopped chicory
  (wet)
2 large garlic cloves, sliced
¼ teaspoon salt
1 teaspoon olive oil

1. To prepare the batter, whisk the flour, baking powder, oregano, salt, and pepper together in a large bowl. Whisk the eggs, whites, milk, and olive oil together in a 2-cup measure. Pour over the dry ingredients in the bowl and stir to mix. (This may be refrigerated, covered, up to 8 hours.) Spoon the batter into a 9-inch square baking pan coated with vegetable oil spray.

2. Preheat the oven to 375°.

3. Place the wet chicory in a medium saucepan. Cover and cook over low heat for 10 minutes until wilted. Remove, drain, squeeze, and cool.

4. Spread the chicory over the batter; top with the garlic slices. Sprinkle with the salt and drizzle with the oil. Bake 45 minutes, or until a toothpick inserted in the center comes out dry.

SERVES 4

**Variation:** Add ⅓ cup hydrated, drained, and chopped sun-dried tomatoes to the batter. Top with cooked, wilted escarole instead of chicory.

**Kilocalories 374 Kc • Protein 16 Gm • Fat 8 Gm • Percent of calories from fat 20%
• Cholesterol 107 mg • Dietary Fiber 9 Gm • Sodium 756 mg • Calcium 448 mg**

# Spinach Crust Pizza with Fresh Tomatoes

*In this recipe the spinach is in the dough rather than on it.*

½ cup warm water (105 to 115°)
1 package active dry yeast
½ teaspoon sugar
2 cups all-purpose flour
¾ teaspoon salt
1 tablespoon olive oil
1 package (10 ounces) frozen
   chopped spinach, thawed,
   drained, and squeezed

*Topping:*

4 medium (about 1 pound) thinly
   sliced ripe tomatoes
¼ teaspoon kosher salt
¼ teaspoon freshly ground
   pepper
1 cup shredded smoked
   mozzarella (about 4 ounces) or
   ⅓ cup grated Romano cheese

1. Pour the water in the bowl of a food processor fitted with the steel blade. Sprinkle with the yeast and sugar. Let it stand for 10 minutes until foamy.

2. Add the flour, salt, and oil to the yeast mixture and pulse 4 or 5 times until combined. Add the spinach and process 20 seconds until a ball forms. Process 30 seconds longer to knead. Knead by hand 1 minute on a floured surface. Place in a large bowl coated with vegetable oil spray, turning to coat. Cover with plastic wrap and let the dough rise for 1 hour.

3. Place the dough in the center of a 12-inch pizza pan coated with vegetable oil spray. Spread to the edges of the pan. Cover with a clean towel and let it stand for 30 minutes until slightly puffed.

4. Preheat the oven to 500°.

5. Arrange the tomatoes on top of the dough; sprinkle with the salt and pepper. Top with the cheese. Bake about 25 minutes until the edges are lightly browned and crisp.

SERVES 6

Kilocalories 253 Kc • Protein 12 Gm • Fat 5 Gm • Percent of calories from fat 18%
• Cholesterol 7 mg • Dietary Fiber 4 Gm • Sodium 530 mg • Calcium 253 mg

# Broccoli Raab, Mushroom, and Olive Pizza

1 pound frozen pizza dough
2 cups sliced fresh mushrooms
1½ tablespoons olive oil
½ teaspoon red pepper flakes

4 cups chopped broccoli raab
  leaves
½ teaspoon salt
10 large black pitted olives,
  chopped

1. Defrost the dough according to the package directions.

2. Combine the mushrooms, ½ tablespoon of the oil, and the red pepper in a large nonstick skillet. Cover and cook over low heat 10 minutes. Increase the heat to medium; add the broccoli raab and salt. Cover again and cook 5 minutes, stirring occasionally.

3. Place the dough in the center of a 12-inch pizza pan coated with vegetable oil spray. Spread to the edges of the pan. Cover with a clean towel and let it stand for 30 minutes until slightly puffed.

4. Preheat the oven to 450°.

5. Spoon the broccoli raab mixture to the edges of the pie. Top with the olives and drizzle with the remaining 1 tablespoon oil. Bake 15 minutes until the edges are golden and crispy.

SERVES 6

Kilocalories 235 Kc • Protein 8 Gm • Fat 7 Gm • Percent of calories from fat 27% • Cholesterol 0 mg • Dietary Fiber 4 Gm • Sodium 774 mg • Calcium 112 mg

# Pizza Shell with Kale, Corn, and Basil-Tomato Feta Cheese

*These ready-made crusts (two to a package) are great in a pinch.*

1 large ready-made pizza shell (with packet of tomato sauce)
1 package (10 ounces) frozen chopped kale, thawed, drained, and squeezed

1 package (10 ounces) frozen corn, thawed and drained
½ cup crumbled feta cheese with basil and tomato (about 2 ounces)

1. Preheat the oven to 450°.
2. Spread the sauce over the shell. Top with the kale and corn. Sprinkle evenly with the cheese. Bake 8 to 10 minutes until browned.

SERVES 6

**Variation:** Spinach Pizza with Pesto-Monterey Jack Cheese: 1½ tablespoons olive oil, 4 cups finely chopped spinach, ¼ teaspoon freshly ground pepper, ½ cup fresh grated pesto-flavored Monterey Jack cheese. Preheat the oven to 450°. Heat the oil in a large nonstick skillet over medium heat. Add the spinach and pepper and cook 2 minutes, stirring frequently. Cool. Spread the spinach over the crust with a fork. Sprinkle with the cheese and bake 8 to 10 minutes.

**Kilocalories 257 Kc • Protein 10 Gm • Fat 5 Gm • Percent of calories from fat 17% • Cholesterol 9 mg • Dietary Fiber 4 Gm • Sodium 734 mg • Calcium 118 mg**

# Broccoli Raab and Anchovy Stromboli

*One day at the supermarket I found a product that I didn't know existed—refrigerator pizza crust in a can, and voilà! Look for it near the refrigerator biscuits.*

1 bunch broccoli raab (about 1¼ pounds), stems removed and leaves coarsely chopped
1 package (10 ounces) refrigerator pizza crust
6 anchovy fillets, finely chopped

2 tablespoons sun-dried tomato bits
¼ teaspoon freshly ground pepper
1 tablespoon olive oil

1. Preheat the oven to 425°.

2. Save the broccoli raab stems for soup or stir-fry. Place the leaves in a collapsible steamer basket set over simmering water in a wide saucepan. Cover and steam 5 to 7 minutes until tender. Drain and cool, then squeeze lightly between paper towels.

3. Unroll the dough and press into a 13 × 11-inch rectangle on a baking sheet coated with vegetable oil spray. Spread the broccoli raab to within 1 inch of the edges; sprinkle with the anchovy, tomatoes, and pepper and drizzle with the oil. Roll up starting at a short end and pinch the ends together to seal (the roll will be approximately 12 inches long). Bake about 18 minutes until browned and crisp. Let it stand 5 minutes before slicing.

SERVES 2

Kilocalories 373 Kc • Protein 13 Gm • Fat 10 Gm • Percent of calories from fat 23% • Cholesterol 7 mg • Dietary Fiber 9 Gm • Sodium 1084 mg • Calcium 280 mg

# Escarole in Puff Pastry

*This is a terrific hot antipasto or side dish.*

1½ tablespoons olive oil
2 tablespoons pignoli nuts
1 large garlic clove, minced
¼ teaspoon red pepper flakes

1 pound escarole, trimmed and
  chopped
¼ teaspoon salt
1 sheet puff pastry, thawed

1. Preheat the oven to 400°.

2. Heat the oil in a large nonstick skillet over medium heat. Add the nuts, garlic, and pepper flakes and cook 1 minute, stirring constantly.

3. Carefully add the wet escarole to the skillet and stir to combine. Cover and cook 10 minutes until tender, stirring frequently. Remove from the heat, uncover, and stir in the salt. Cool.

4. Roll the puff pastry sheet on a lightly floured surface to a 14 × 10-inch rectangle. Spread the escarole mixture to within 1 inch of the edge. Roll up, starting at one long edge, jelly-roll fashion, and pinch the ends together to seal. Carefully lift onto the baking sheet with a large spatula. Bake 30 minutes. Let it stand 10 minutes before slicing.

SERVES 4

Kilocalories 156 Kc • Protein 4 Gm • Fat 12 Gm • Percent of calories from fat 67%
• Cholesterol 0 mg • Dietary Fiber 4 Gm • Sodium 200 mg • Calcium 63 mg

# Low-Fat Mustard Green Biscuits

4 cups coarsely chopped fresh
   mustard greens
2¼ cups low-fat biscuit mix

½ teaspoon salt
¾ cup plus 1 tablespoon skim
   milk

1. Preheat the oven to 400°.

2. Place the greens in a collapsible steamer basket set over simmering water in a wide saucepan. Cover and steam 10 minutes. Carefully lift the basket and place in the sink to cool. Place the greens in a clean kitchen towel and squeeze out any excess liquid. Chop finely.

3. Combine the greens, 2 cups of the biscuit mix, and the salt in a large bowl. Gradually stir in ¾ cup milk until a soft dough forms. Turn the dough onto a lightly floured surface. Flour your hands and pat the dough into a ½-inch thickness, sprinkling with the remaining ¼ cup biscuit mix if it is too sticky to handle. Cut out rounds with a 2-inch cutter and place close together on a baking sheet coated with vegetable oil spray. Brush the biscuits with the remaining 1 tablespoon skim milk. Bake 15 to 18 minutes until lightly browned. Serve immediately.

MAKES 16 BISCUITS

Kilocalories 78 Kc • Protein 2 Gm • Fat 3 Gm • Percent of calories from fat 30% • Cholesterol 0 mg • Dietary Fiber 1 Gm • Sodium 296 mg • Calcium 55 mg

# Savory Spinach and Onion Pancakes

2 teaspoons vegetable oil
¼ cup finely chopped onion
2 cups finely chopped fresh
  spinach
1 cup low-fat biscuit mix

½ teaspoon salt
½ cup skim milk
1 large egg, lightly beaten
1 tablespoon whipped butter at
  room temperature, optional

1. Heat the oil in a medium skillet over medium heat. Add the onion and cook 30 seconds. Add the spinach and cook 3 minutes, stirring frequently.

2. Combine the biscuit mix and salt in a medium bowl. Stir in the milk, egg, and spinach mixture until the batter is fairly smooth.

3. Preheat a griddle or large nonstick skillet over medium heat. Coat with vegetable oil spray. Pour a scant ¼ cup pancake batter onto the griddle and cook each pancake about 1½ minutes on each side until lightly browned and puffed. Serve immediately with butter, if desired.

SERVES 4 (MAKES 8 PANCAKES)

Kilocalories 188 Kc • Protein 6 Gm • Fat 8 Gm • Percent of calories from fat 39% • Cholesterol 54 mg • Dietary Fiber 2 Gm • Sodium 727 mg • Calcium 128 mg

# Alsatian Tart

*This recipe was inspired by four-star chef Jean-Georges Vongerichten, whose restaurant JO JO in Manhattan serves fabulous French bistro food prepared with juices, vegetable broths, flavored oils, and vinaigrettes—a lighter touch for today's modern cuisine. Serve this tart as an appetizer or side dish.*

2 cups finely shredded cabbage
½ cup thinly sliced onion
1 large garlic clove, minced
1 tablespoon vegetable oil
¼ teaspoon salt

¼ teaspoon freshly ground pepper
¼ cup shredded Gruyère or Swiss cheese
2 tablespoons nonfat sour cream
4 sheets phyllo dough

1. Preheat the oven to 400°.

2. Combine the cabbage, onion, garlic, oil, salt, and pepper in a large nonstick skillet. Cover, and cook over medium-low heat 10 minutes. Uncover, and cook 10 minutes longer, stirring frequently until just browned. Remove from the heat, cool slightly, and stir in the cheese and sour cream.

3. While the cabbage mixture is cooking, stack the phyllo sheets. Cut into an 8-inch round (use an 8-inch cake pan inverted onto the phyllo and cut around the rim). Spray a 9-inch circle on a baking sheet. Place one sheet of phyllo onto the coated surface. Coat the phyllo with oil spray and repeat with the remaining phyllo sheets until stacked again. Bake 5 minutes; turn carefully with a spatula, and bake 3 minutes longer.

4. Spread the cabbage mixture evenly over the phyllo. Bake 8 to 10 minutes until the top is lightly browned. Cut into wedges and serve immediately.

SERVES 4

Kilocalories 140 Kc • Protein 5 Gm • Fat 7 Gm • Percent of calories from fat 42% • Cholesterol 7 mg • Dietary Fiber 1 Gm • Sodium 269 mg • Calcium 103 mg

# 11

# Sweet Ending

I am sure you will be tempted to believe that this is a fantasy tart—a real stretch to use greens in a dessert. But this tart is not the product of an overactive imagination. I tasted one exactly like it in Lucca, an ancient walled city in the Tuscan hills of Italy. Heavily spiced, this tart may have its origins in the Renaissance period (beginning in the fourteenth century). During this time, sweet and savory combinations in food were common.

Always on the lookout for anything unusual in the food department, I entered this new taste sensation in my travel journal. Six months later, I began this book and was delighted to be able to end on an authentic sweet note. The recipe is not low in fat, but tastes just the way I remember it. If you're feeling adventurous, top each slice with a mound of freshly whipped sweet cream!

# Torta di Verdura (Sweet Greens Tart)

*Crust:*

2½ cups all-purpose flour
⅓ cup sugar
½ teaspoon baking powder
¼ teaspoon salt
8 tablespoons (1 stick) chilled
   unsalted butter, cut into pieces
1 large egg
¼ cup whole milk
½ teaspoon vanilla extract

*Filling:*

2 pounds Swiss chard (or green
   of choice), stems removed
1 cup whole milk
¼ cup sugar
3 tablespoons all-purpose flour
2 large eggs
1 egg yolk
1 teaspoon grated orange zest
½ teaspoon ground cinnamon
¼ teaspoon ground allspice
¼ teaspoon grated nutmeg
¼ cup finely chopped candied
   fruit
¼ cup chopped walnuts

1. To prepare the crust, combine the flour, sugar, baking powder, and salt in a large bowl. Blend in the butter with a pastry blender or fork, until the mixture resembles coarse meal. Add the egg, milk, and vanilla extract. Toss with a fork until the dough holds together. Squeeze the dough together and shape into a disk. Cut the dough into thirds and flatten one-third into a disk and shape the remaining two-thirds into another disk. Wrap each in plastic wrap and refrigerate at least 1 hour or up to 2 days.

2. Place the chard leaves in a collapsible steamer basket set over simmering water in a wide saucepan. Cover and steam 15 minutes, until wilted. Cool, then wrap the chard in a clean kitchen towel and squeeze out the excess liquid. Finely chop the chard and place it in a medium mixing bowl. Stir in the remaining filling ingredients and set aside.

3. Place the oven rack on the lowest level. Preheat the oven to 350°.

4. Roll out the larger piece of dough on a lightly floured surface, to an 11-inch circle. Press the dough into a 9-inch fluted tart pan with removable bottom. Trim. Cover and refrigerate 30 minutes.

5. Roll out the remaining disk to a 10-inch circle, and with a fluted pastry wheel, cut it into ½-inch-wide strips. Pour the filling into the pre-

pared tart shell. Place the strips about an inch apart over the filling, forming a lattice pattern. Press the ends against the sides of the tart shell to seal.

6. Bake about 1 hour and 10 minutes or until the tart is puffy and golden brown. Let it cool on a wire rack 30 minutes. Remove the rim and cool completely before serving.

SERVES 8

Kilocalories 434 Kc • Protein 11 Gm • Fat 18 Gm • Percent of calories from fat 37% • Cholesterol 117 mg • Dietary Fiber 3 Gm • Sodium 392 mg • Calcium 139 mg

# Bibliography

Arkin, Frieda. *The Complete Book of Kitchen Wisdom*. New York: Henry Holt & Company, Inc., 1993.

Ballentye, Janet. *Joy of Gardening Cookbook*. New York: Garden Way, Inc., 1984.

Belk, Sarah. *Around the Southern Table*. New York: Simon & Schuster, 1991.

*Betty Crocker's Cookbook*. New York: Golden Press, 1988.

Claiborne, Craig. *The New York Times International Cookbook*. New York: Harper & Row, 1971.

Clingerman, Polly. *The Kitchen Companion*. Gaithersburg, Md.: The American Cooking Guild, 1994.

Cunningham, Marion. *The Fannie Farmer Cookbook*. New York: Alfred A. Knopf, 1990.

Della Croce, Julia. *The Little Dishes of Italy: Antipasti*. San Francisco: Chronicle Books, 1993.

Gethers, Judy. *The Sandwich Book*. New York: Random House, 1990.

Hazen, Giuliano. *The Classic Pasta Cookbook*. New York: Dorling Kindersley, Inc., 1993.

Hazen, Janet. *The Sophisticated Sandwich*. Berkeley: Aris Books, 1989.

Herbst, Sharon Tyler. *Food Lover's Companion*. New York: Barron's, 1990.

Kasper, Lynn Rosetto. *The Splendid Table*. New York: William Morrow, Inc., 1992.

Leahy, Linda Romanelli. *The Oat Bran Cookbook*. New York: Fawcett Gold Medal, 1989.

Long, Kathi. *Mexican Light Cooking*. New York: The Putnam Publishing Group, 1992.

MacMillian, Norma. *The Cook's Kitchen Bible*. New York: Smithmark Publishers Inc., 1995.

McCune, Kelly. *Grill Book*. New York: Harper & Row, 1989.

McGee, Harold. *On Food and Cooking*. New York: Charles Scribner's Sons, 1984.

Morash, Marion. *The Victory Garden Cookbook*. New York: Alfred A. Knopf, 1982.

Riely, Elizabeth. *The Chef's Companion*. New York: Van Nostrand Reinhold Company, 1986.

Routhier, Nicole. *Cooking Under Wraps*. New York: William Morrow, Inc., 1993.

Scicolone, Michele. *The Antipasto Table*. New York: William Morrow, Inc., 1991.

Scott, Sally Anne. *For the Love of Vegetables*. Santa Rosa, Ca.: ColeGroup, 1994.

Simmons, Marie. *The Light Touch Cookbook*. Shelburne, Vt.: Chapters Publishing Ltd., 1992.

Stallworth, Lyn, and Kennedy, Rod, Jr. *The Country Fair Cookbook*. New York: Hyperion, 1994.

Street, Myra. (Edited and Adapted) *La Cucina*. London: Orbis Book Publishing, 1986.

Toussaint-Samat, Maguelonne. *History of Food*. Cambridge, Mass.: Blackwell Publishers, 1992.

Vongerichten, Jean-Georges. *Simple Cuisine*. New York: Prentice-Hall Press, 1990.

Zimmerman, Linda, and Gilliland, Gerri. *Grills & Greens*. New York: Clarkson N. Potter, Inc., 1993.

# Index